Green Synthesis of Nanomaterials and Their Biological Applications

Green Synthesis of Nanomaterials and Their Biological Applications

Editor

Giovanni Benelli

MDPI • Basel • Beijing • Wuhan • Barcelona • Belgrade • Manchester • Tokyo • Cluj • Tianjin

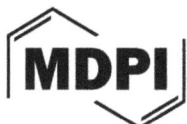

Editor
Giovanni Benelli
Agriculture, Food and
Environment
University of Pisa
Pisa
Italy

Editorial Office
MDPI
St. Alban-Anlage 66
4052 Basel, Switzerland

This is a reprint of articles from the Special Issue published online in the open access journal *Nanomaterials* (ISSN 2079-4991) (available at: www.mdpi.com/journal/nanomaterials/special_issues/Nano_insecticides).

For citation purposes, cite each article independently as indicated on the article page online and as indicated below:

LastName, A.A.; LastName, B.B.; LastName, C.C. Article Title. *Journal Name* **Year**, *Volume Number*, Page Range.

ISBN 978-3-0365-3185-4 (Hbk)
ISBN 978-3-0365-3184-7 (PDF)

© 2022 by the authors. Articles in this book are Open Access and distributed under the Creative Commons Attribution (CC BY) license, which allows users to download, copy and build upon published articles, as long as the author and publisher are properly credited, which ensures maximum dissemination and a wider impact of our publications.

The book as a whole is distributed by MDPI under the terms and conditions of the Creative Commons license CC BY-NC-ND.

Contents

About the Editor vii

Preface to "Green Synthesis of Nanomaterials and Their Biological Applications" ix

Giovanni Benelli
Green Synthesis of Nanomaterials and Their Biological Applications
Reprinted from: *Nanomaterials* **2021**, *11*, 2842, doi:10.3390/nano11112842 1

Marta Fiedot-Toboła, Anna Dmochowska, Bartłomiej Potaniec, Joanna Czajkowska, Roman Jedrzejewski and Magdalena Wilk-Kozubek et al.
Gallic Acid Based Black Tea Extract as a Stabilizing Agent in ZnO Particles Green Synthesis
Reprinted from: *Nanomaterials* **2021**, *11*, 1816, doi:10.3390/nano11071816 3

Kaushik Kumar Bharadwaj, Bijuli Rabha, Siddhartha Pati, Bhabesh Kumar Choudhury, Tanmay Sarkar and Sonit Kumar Gogoi et al.
Green Synthesis of Silver Nanoparticles Using *Diospyros malabarica* Fruit Extract and Assessments of Their Antimicrobial, Anticancer and Catalytic Reduction of 4-Nitrophenol (4-NP)
Reprinted from: *Nanomaterials* **2021**, *11*, 1999, doi:10.3390/nano11081999 21

Paraskevi Agrafioti, Sofia Faliagka, Evagelia Lampiri, Merle Orth, Mark Pätzel and Nikolaos Katsoulas et al.
Evaluation of Silica-Coated Insect Proof Nets for the Control of *Aphis fabae, Sitophilus oryzae*, and *Tribolium confusum*
Reprinted from: *Nanomaterials* **2020**, *10*, 1658, doi:10.3390/nano10091658 45

Giovanni Benelli, Lucia Pavoni, Valeria Zeni, Renato Ricciardi, Francesca Cosci and Gloria Cacopardo et al.
Developing a Highly Stable *Carlina acaulis* Essential Oil Nanoemulsion for Managing *Lobesia botrana*
Reprinted from: *Nanomaterials* **2020**, *10*, 1867, doi:10.3390/nano10091867 57

Jitong Zhong, Xiaocan Xu and Yu-Sheng Lin
Tunable Terahertz Metamaterial with Electromagnetically Induced Transparency Characteristic for Sensing Application
Reprinted from: *Nanomaterials* **2021**, *11*, 2175, doi:10.3390/nano11092175 73

Huiliang Ou, Fangyuan Lu, Zefeng Xu and Yu-Sheng Lin
Terahertz Metamaterial with Multiple Resonances for Biosensing Application
Reprinted from: *Nanomaterials* **2020**, *10*, 1038, doi:10.3390/nano10061038 85

Aishah E. Albalawi, Abdullah D. Alanazi, Parastoo Baharvand, Maryam Sepahvand and Hossein Mahmoudvand
High Potency of Organic and Inorganic Nanoparticles to Treat Cystic Echinococcosis: An Evidence-Based Review
Reprinted from: *Nanomaterials* **2020**, *10*, 2538, doi:10.3390/nano10122538 97

About the Editor

Giovanni Benelli

Giovanni Benelli serves as Associate Professor of General and Applied Entomology at the Department of Agriculture, Food and Environment, University of Pisa, Italy. He teaches Agrarian Zoology, Biological Control, Trends and Challenges in the Management of Vineyard Pests, and Biotechnologies for Managing Animal Parasites.

He obtained an International Ph.D. in Agrarian and Veterinary Sciences at University of Pisa and Sant'Anna School of Advanced Studies. Giovanni has worked in several international institutions, including University of Hawaii at Manoa (USA) and University of Jaén (Spain).

Giovanni's research focuses on insect behaviour, biological control, chemical ecology (with special reference to sex pheromones and mating disruption), and insect-inspired robotics, covering agricultural pests, as well as vectors of medical and veterinary importance.

He has cooperated with a wide number of researchers worldwide on various research projects (e.g., iGuess-MED PRIMA, STRADIOL). He is actively engaged in third mission activities, through agricultural extension services focused on IPM and biological control of olive and vineyard insect pests.

Giovanni serves as Editor in Chief/Associate Editor/Editorial Board Member for many top-ranked international journals in the field of general and applied entomology.

He has been awarded with various research prizes from international and national organizations, including the Odile Bain Memorial Prize 2018 (Parasites and Vectors & Boehringer Animal Health) and the Antico Fattore Prize 2016 (Accademia dei Georgofili, Firenze). He has been appointed as a Member of Accademia dei Georgofili in December 2021.

Preface to "Green Synthesis of Nanomaterials and Their Biological Applications"

Developing effective products to fight pests and parasites is a key challenge for entomology and parasitology. Despite the relevant amount of research on the "green"insecticides, acaricides, and antiparasitics, mainly covering products of microbial and botanical origin, their practical use in real-world conditions remains limited. This is often due to lack of prolonged efficacy and challenging regulations. Thus, nanotechnologies are currently considered a major option to improve the efficacy and stability of both classic and green insecticides, repellents and antiparasitic drugs, relying to various nanocarriers, including nanoencapsulation and nanoemulsions.

In this scenario, the present book offers novel research insights recently published as a part of the Nanomaterials Special Issue Green Synthesis of Nanomaterials and Their Biological Applications, with the aim to provide an updated overview on the green synthesis of nanomaterials as well as on their possible practical uses in the fields of entomology, parasitology, biomedicine, and environmental research.

Giovanni Benelli
Editor

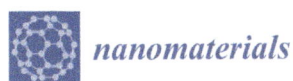

Editorial

Green Synthesis of Nanomaterials and Their Biological Applications

Giovanni Benelli

Department of Agriculture, Food and Environment, University of Pisa, Via del Borghetto 80, 56124 Pisa, Italy; giovanni.benelli@unipi.it; Tel.: +39-050-221-6141

Introduction

Nanomaterials possess valuable physical and chemical properties, which may make them excellent candidates for the development of new insecticides, acaricides, fungicides, drugs, catalysts, and sensors, to cite just some key categories. To avoid the utilization of toxic or high-energy inputs, which are routinely used in nano-synthesis, the "green synthesis" concept has been proposed, outlining the use of microbial-, animal-, and plant-borne compounds as reducing and stabilizing agents. Even though a large number of studies have been published on the topic, many potential applications of nanomaterials have scarcely been explored, and their real-world applications are poorly implemented. This is often due to a lack of prolonged efficacy of the bioactive compounds and challenging regulations. Nanotechnologies are currently considered a strategic option to improve the efficacy and stability of classic and green insecticides, acaricides, repellents and antiparasitic drugs, relying on various nanocarriers, including nanoencapsulation and nanoemulsions.

In this framework, the journal *Nanomaterials* has already dedicated a successful Special Issue to the topic "Green Synthesis of Nanomaterials" in 2019 [1].

The Special Issue "Green Synthesis of Nanomaterials and Their Biological Applications" represents a continuation of the former, with another collection of top-quality articles in this research area. Particular attention has been devoted to entomological research, because the widespread overuse of synthetic insecticides leads to the rapid development of resistance in target species, and non-target effects on human health and the environment. A comparable scenario is well recognized in parasitology concerning the use of drugs to manage parasites of public health importance.

Herein, both original research and reviews have been considered for publication. The present Special Issue includes contributions on the following research topics:

(i) Green-based processes improving the stability of nanomaterials [2];
(ii) The development of green synthesis protocols for the preparation of nanomaterials with antibacterial and anticancer activity, as well as acting as catalytic reductors of nitrophenols [3];
(iii) The development of novel insecticides against key insect pests, including highly stable insecticidal nanoemulsions toxic to moth larvae [4], as well as silica-nanoparticle-coated insecticidal nets effective against aphids and stored-product beetles [5];
(iv) The development of new terahertz metamaterials for biosensing applications [6,7].

The Special Issue ends with a review on cystic echinococcosis [8], a dangerous and hard-to-manage parasitic disease [9,10], summarizing current knowledge on the scolicidal activity of organic and inorganic nanoparticles evaluated through in vitro, in vivo, and ex vivo studies, also considering possible synergistic effects with anti-parasitic drugs currently used.

Overall, I am grateful to all the authors for their fine contributions to the present Special Issue, and hope that the published studies will pave the way for novel real-world applications of green nanomaterials.

Funding: This article received no external funding.

Data Availability Statement: Not applicable.

Acknowledgments: I am grateful to Cassie Zhang for her kind assistance in the organization of this Special Issue.

Conflicts of Interest: The author declares no conflict of interest.

References

1. Benelli, G. Green Synthesis of Nanomaterials. *Nanomaterials* **2019**, *9*, 1275. [CrossRef] [PubMed]
2. Fiedot-Toboła, M.; Dmochowska, A.; Potaniec, B.; Czajkowska, J.; Jędrzejewski, R.; Wilk-Kozubek, M.; Carolak, E.; Cybińska, J. Gallic Acid Based Black Tea Extract as a Stabilizing Agent in ZnO Particles Green Synthesis. *Nanomaterials* **2021**, *11*, 1816. [CrossRef] [PubMed]
3. Bharadwaj, K.K.; Rabha, B.; Pati, S.; Choudhury, B.K.; Sarkar, T.; Gogoi, S.K.; Kakati, N.; Baishya, D.; Kari, Z.A.; Edinur, H.A. Green Synthesis of Silver Nanoparticles Using *Diospyros malabarica* Fruit Extract and Assessments of Their Antimicrobial, Anticancer and Catalytic Reduction of 4-Nitrophenol (4-NP). *Nanomaterials* **2021**, *11*, 1999. [CrossRef] [PubMed]
4. Benelli, G.; Pavoni, L.; Zeni, V.; Ricciardi, R.; Cosci, F.; Cacopardo, G.; Gendusa, S.; Spinozzi, E.; Petrelli, R.; Cappellacci, L.; et al. Developing a Highly Stable *Carlina acaulis* Essential Oil Nanoemulsion for Managing *Lobesia botrana*. *Nanomaterials* **2020**, *10*, 1867. [CrossRef] [PubMed]
5. Agrafioti, P.; Faliagka, S.; Lampiri, E.; Orth, M.; Pätzel, M.; Katsoulas, N.; Athanassiou, C.G. Evaluation of Silica-Coated Insect Proof Nets for the Control of *Aphis fabae*, *Sitophilus oryzae*, and *Tribolium confusum*. *Nanomaterials* **2020**, *10*, 1658. [CrossRef] [PubMed]
6. Ou, H.; Lu, F.; Xu, Z.; Lin, Y.-S. Terahertz Metamaterial with Multiple Resonances for Biosensing Application. *Nanomaterials* **2020**, *10*, 1038. [CrossRef] [PubMed]
7. Zhong, J.; Xu, X.; Lin, Y.-S. Tunable Terahertz Metamaterial with Electromagnetically Induced Transparency Characteristic for Sensing Application. *Nanomaterials* **2021**, *11*, 2175. [CrossRef] [PubMed]
8. Albalawi, A.E.; Alanazi, A.D.; Baharvand, P.; Sepahvand, M.; Mahmoudvand, H. High Potency of Organic and Inorganic Nanoparticles to Treat Cystic Echinococcosis: An Evidence-Based Review. *Nanomaterials* **2020**, *10*, 2538. [CrossRef] [PubMed]
9. Benelli, G.; Wassermann, M.; Brattig, N.W. Insects dispersing taeniid eggs: Who and how? *Vet. Parasitol.* **2021**, *295*, 109450. [CrossRef] [PubMed]
10. Larrieu, E.; Gavidia, C.M.; Lightowlers, M.W. Control of cystic echinococcosis: Background and prospects. *Zoonoses Public Health* **2019**, *66*, 889–899. [CrossRef] [PubMed]

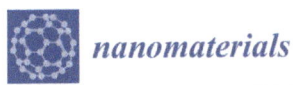

Article

Gallic Acid Based Black Tea Extract as a Stabilizing Agent in ZnO Particles Green Synthesis

Marta Fiedot-Toboła [1,*], Anna Dmochowska [1], Bartłomiej Potaniec [1], Joanna Czajkowska [1], Roman Jędrzejewski [1], Magdalena Wilk-Kozubek [1], Ewa Carolak [1] and Joanna Cybińska [1,2]

1 Łukasiewicz Research Network—PORT Polish Center for Technology Development, Stabłowicka 147, 54-066 Wrocław, Poland; anna.dmochowska@ensam.eu (A.D.); bartlomiej.potaniec@port.lukasiewicz.gov.pl (B.P.); joanna.czajkowska@port.lukasiewicz.gov.pl (J.C.); roman.jedrzejewski@port.lukasiewicz.gov.pl (R.J.); magdalena.wilk-kozubek@port.lukasiewicz.gov.pl (M.W.-K.); ewa.carolak@port.lukasiewicz.gov.pl (E.C.); joanna.cybinska@port.lukasiewicz.gov.pl (J.C.)
2 Faculty of Chemistry, University of Wrocław, 14 F. Joliot-Curie Str., 50-383 Wrocław, Poland
* Correspondence: marta.fiedot-tobola@port.lukasiewicz.gov.pl; Tel.: +48-717-347-154

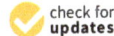

Citation: Fiedot-Toboła, M.; Dmochowska, A.; Potaniec, B.; Czajkowska, J.; Jędrzejewski, R.; Wilk-Kozubek, M.; Carolak, E.; Cybińska, J. Gallic Acid Based Black Tea Extract as a Stabilizing Agent in ZnO Particles Green Synthesis. *Nanomaterials* **2021**, *11*, 1816. https://doi.org/10.3390/nano11071816

Academic Editor: Giovanni Benelli

Received: 22 June 2021
Accepted: 9 July 2021
Published: 13 July 2021

Publisher's Note: MDPI stays neutral with regard to jurisdictional claims in published maps and institutional affiliations.

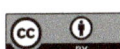

Copyright: © 2021 by the authors. Licensee MDPI, Basel, Switzerland. This article is an open access article distributed under the terms and conditions of the Creative Commons Attribution (CC BY) license (https://creativecommons.org/licenses/by/4.0/).

Abstract: In this work, zinc oxide particles (ZnO NPs) green synthesis with the application of black tea extract (BT) is presented. A thorough investigation of the properties of the extract and the obtained materials was conducted by using Fourier transform infrared spectroscopy (FTIR), liquid chromatography-mass spectrometry (LC-MS), X-ray diffraction (XRD), scanning electron microscopy (SEM), thermogravimetric analysis (TGA), and quadrupole mass spectroscopy (QMS). The obtained results indicated that the amount of used BT strongly influenced the morphology, chemical, and crystalline structure of the obtained particles. The investigation demonstrated that the substance present in black tea (BT) extract, which was adsorbed on the ZnO surface, was in fact gallic acid. It was found that gallic acid controls the crystallization process of ZnO by temporarily blocking the zinc cations. Additionally, these organic molecules interact with the hydroxide group of the precipitant. This blocks the dehydration process stabilizing the zinc hydroxide forms and hinders its transformation into zinc oxide. Performed measurements indicated that obtained ZnO particles have great antioxidant and antimicrobial properties, which are significantly correlated with ZnO–gallic acid interactions.

Keywords: zinc oxide; nanoparticles; black tea extract; gallic acid; green synthesis; antioxidants; antimicrobial activity

1. Introduction

Biosynthesis, or green synthesis of nanoparticles, has been under the radar of many researchers. The various methods following the principles of green chemistry have received a lot of attention due to the low-toxicity of used substrates, their affordability, and inexpensiveness [1]. Metal or metal oxide nanostructures have been synthesized with an application of various extracts prepared from the part of a plant. The extracts are used as either stabilizing or reducing agents. Some of the methods involve using the leaves of plants such as jackfruit (*Artocarpus heterophyllus*) [2] or *Carissa carandas* [3], flowers like *Anchusa italica* [4], the fruits of plants, including *Acacia nilotica* [5], the peels of the fruits (e.g., a banana (*Musa paradisiaca*) peel [6]), or the root of the plant like *Berberis vulgaris* [7].

Among many nanomaterials, zinc oxide nanostructures are exceptionally attractive thanks to their unique functional properties and the diversity of their applications. They have been used in many fields as gas sensors [8], piezoelectric devices [9], solar cells [10], fillers in polymeric nanocomposites [11,12], coatings [13,14], antimicrobial agents [15], and in textiles [16].

Tea infusion is one of the most popular beverages worldwide. The brew is prepared from the leaves of the *Camellia sinensis* plant, which originally comes from China [17].

Depending on the processing of the leaves, the types of tea may be divided into three major groups—green, oolong, and black tea, all of them varying in the fermentation level of the leaves [18]. Green tea is the unfermented one, black tea is completely fermented, while oolong tea stands in the middle, being only partially fermented [19].

The leading components found in tea are polyphenols, which account for 20–35% of dry weight [20]. The fermentation process causes changes in the amount of polyphenols in the leaves due to their oxidative polymerization, leading to the formation of thearubigins and theaflavins, which are responsible for the dark red color of the black tea [21,22]. The polyphenol group is divided into two main categories of components. The first one being the catechins like (−)-epigallocatechin gallate (EGCG), which can constitute for 50–80% of all the catechins in tea. The second group includes the phenolic acids like gallic acid, whose amount is notably increased in black tea due to the processes occurring during fermentation [23,24].

It was reported that except for polyphenols, tea infusions contain many compounds such as polysaccharides, whose amount depends on the maturity of the tea leaf [25]; alkaloids, with caffeine being the easiest one to find in all kinds of tea [26]; amino acids, with theanine taking up to 50% of all free amino acids found in teas [27]; and saponins that have displayed antifungal activity against *Rhizopus stolonifer* [28]. The amount of the various phytochemicals in the leaves is strongly dependent on the processing during the production, the age of the plant, and its origin. In addition, it is difficult to assess the number and nature of the compounds in the tea infusion as it fluctuates with the preparation method (e.g., brewing time) [29].

The leaves of black tea have been used before in order to obtain various metal or metal oxides nanoparticles. The aqueous extract was employed for synthesizing nanoparticles of palladium [30], iron oxide [31], copper oxide [32], and iron, copper, and silver [33]. In most cases, the black tea extract serves as a reducing agent for the precursor of the nanoparticles. In addition, an ethanol black tea extract was applied for the synthesis of gold nanoparticles [34]. Zinc oxide nanoparticles were also synthesized with black tea extract. Therein, the black tea extract served as the reducing agent for hydrothermal syntheses (e.g., to reduce zinc nitrate [35–37] or zinc sulfate [38]).

In the presented work, zinc oxide structures were successfully obtained by a green synthesis method in which the black tea water extract was used as a stabilizing agent. This natural compound has not been previously used in this role. Due to the complicated composition of the extract and the ability to stabilize the nanoparticles by its individual ingredients, understanding the mechanism of ZnO formation under these conditions is a very difficult scientific issue. Its explanation was the main subject of this article. Moreover, a very important aspect of this work was the analysis of the relationship between the material properties of the obtained nanoparticles and their possible functionality. Therefore, at first, the chemical composition of the black tea extract was characterized. Then, the chemical and crystalline structure, and morphology of the final materials were thoroughly described and compared with the antioxidant and antimicrobial properties of the synthesized ZnO.

2. Materials and Methods

2.1. Black Tea Extract (BT) Preparation

A total of 3.00 g of black tea leaves (purchased at the local grocery store) were weighed in a beaker and mixed with 100 mL of distilled water. The mixture was boiled for approximately 5 min at 100 °C (until the color of the extract turned to a very dark burgundy). The mixture was then cooled down and filtered three times. The black tea extract was stored in a refrigerator at 4 °C until further use.

2.2. Zinc Oxide Particles Synthesis

Various volumes of the black tea extract were added to the 1 M zinc acetate water solution. The goal was to obtain mixtures with the different ratios (v:v) of the black tea extract versus Zn^{2+} ions as follows: 1:12 (BT1), 1:6 (BT2), and 1:1 (BT3). The solutions were mixed with a magnetic stirrer at room temperature for 10 min. Next, the 1.0 M water solution of sodium hydroxide was added dropwise until the pH increased to 12. The obtained suspensions were left to mix for another 2 h at room temperature. Afterward, the precipitants were washed twice with distilled water and centrifuged (20 min, 6000 rpm/4427 rcf). The washing and centrifuging process was repeated twice. The products were dried at 60 °C for about 24 h until constant mass and ground using a mortar. All reagents were purchased from Sigma-Aldrich (Sigma-Aldrich Co., St. Louis, MO, USA).

2.3. Characterization of Black Tea Extract

The chemical composition of the obtained black tea extract was examined by two methods: Fourier transform infrared spectroscopy and liquid chromatography-mass spectrometry.

The FTIR analysis of the functional groups was performed on the dried extract—after water evaporation in 60 °C until constant mass. The sample was ground, mixed with dried spectroscopic grade KBr, and formed into a pellet. The spectrum was recorded in the range of 350–4000 cm^{-1} at 4 cm^{-1} resolution (Tensor 27 EQ spectrometer, Bruker, Bremen, Germany).

LC-MS analysis was executed as follows: right before the measurement, 200 µL of the extract was diluted to 1 mL with ultrapure water and used for LC injection. Hypergrade (LC-MS grade) solvents were used. The calibration mixture was 10 mM NaOH in 1:1 (v:v) water:isopropanol with the addition of 0.2% formic acid. The measurement was performed on high-resolution Q-ToF spectrometer maXis impact (Bruker Daltonics, Bremen, Germany) equipped with an electrospray ionization (ESI) source and connected to a Dionex Ulti-Mate 3000 RSLC (Thermo Scientific, Waltham, MA, USA) ultrahigh-performance liquid chromatograph. The chromatographic separations were carried out on Syncronis C18 100.00 × 2.10 mm × 1.70 µm column (Thermo Scientific, Waltham, MA, USA). All reagents were purchased from Sigma-Aldrich (Sigma-Aldrich Co., St. Louis, MO, USA). The data were analyzed with Data Analysis 4.1 software (Thermo Scientific, Waltham, MA, USA). The extracted ion chromatograms (EICs) for every ion that gave good quality fragment spectrum were generated semi-automatically with a manual check of every chromatographic peak generated that way. For each EIC peak, the molecular formula of the parent ion was generated using the SmartFormula algorithm with maximum admissible error of 5 ppm (10 ppm in case of no valid formulas in 5 ppm range). Then, MS/MS spectra for every EIC peak were compared against METLIN and NIST 11 spectral databases. For every compound identified that way, a specific record was created. In the case of most of the chromatographic peaks, we were not able to get a clear hit on the database, so we used literature data on tea extract analysis for manual identification of certain compounds based on retention order, fragment spectra comparison, etc. [39,40]. For the remaining peaks that were not identified by the database and literature search, we performed manual fragment spectra annotation and came up with the most probable identification or partial identification.

2.4. Characterization of ZnO Particles

The X-ray diffraction analysis (Empyrean, Malvern PANalytical, Malvern, UK) was performed to determinate the phase composition, crystallite size, and strain. The following parameters were set: Cu-Kα radiation (λ = 1.54 Å), operating voltage—40 kV, current 30 mA, 2Θ range 10–100°, step 0.007°, scan speed 150 s/step (Pixcel detector). The X'Pert HighScore Plus program with ICDD PDF-4+ 2019 database was used to identify the phase composition of the samples. The zinc oxide crystallite size and lattice strain were calculated by using a line profile analysis (LPA in HighScore Plus, Malvern PANalytical, Malvern, UK) according to the Williamson–Hall method (1) [41].

$$\beta_{hkl}\cos(\theta) = \frac{k\lambda}{D} + 4\varepsilon\sin \tag{1}$$

where β is the peak width at half maximum (FWHM) [rad]; k is the Scherrer constant (0.9); λ is the wavelength of Cu-Kα radiation; D is the crystallite size; and ε is the lattice strain.

The morphology of the ZnO powders was determined by scanning electron microscopy analysis (SEM) using a dual beam microscope (Helios 450HP, Nanolab Technologies Inc, Milpitas, CA, USA). The samples were placed directly on a carbon tape without coatings and imaged at a low-voltage mode (≤5 keV). The approximation of the obtained particle dimensions was based on dimensioning from a series of SEM images and their averaging.

The FTIR spectroscopy was used to analyze the functional groups in the materials. The measurement parameters were the same as for the analysis of the black tea extract.

Thermogravimetric analysis was performed to determine the powders' thermal stability (TGA2 thermogravimetric analyzer, Mettler Toledo, Columbus, OH, USA). The measurements were conducted using alumina crucibles (~5.00 mg) in an air atmosphere (30 mL/min) in the range of 25–600 °C with a 10 °C/min heating rate. Additionally, the Vyazovkin free kinetics model (2) [42] was used to determine the activation energy (E_a) of the degradation process. For this purpose, the TG measurements were repeated in the same conditions but with different heating rates (5, 15, 20 °C/min).

$$\frac{d\alpha}{dt} = A\exp\left(\frac{-E}{RT}\right) f(\alpha) \tag{2}$$

where R is the gas constant; a is the slope of linear plot; t is the time; a is the constant; T is the temperature.

The analysis of the gases evolved during the decomposition of the ZnO particles was done by using the STA 449 F1 Jupiter Netzsch thermal analyzer coupled with a quadrupole mass spectrometer QMS Aëlos 403D (Netzsch, Selb, Germany) and Tensor 27 EQ spectrophotometer (Bruker, Bremen, Germany). The sample that was synthesized with the largest amount of black tea extract was heated up to 600 °C with the rate of 10 °C/min in the nitrogen atmosphere (50 mL/min).

The antioxidant capacity of the black tea extract and ZnO particles was determined using the 2,2'-azino-bis(3-ethylbenzothiazoline-6-sulfonic acid (ABTS) assay. This spectrophotometric assay is based on the ability of the antioxidant substance to quench the colored free ABTS radical cation [43]. The blue-green colored ABTS radical cation, formed by the direct reaction of ABTS with potassium persulfate, has absorption maxima at 415, 645, 734, and 815 nm. The quenching of the free ABTS radical cation results in a decrease in absorbance at the selected wavelength, which was visualized by discoloration of the ABTS radical cation. The degree of discoloration of the ABTS radical cation measured over time depends on the concentration of the antioxidant substance and the duration of the reaction, so that for a fixed reaction time, the antioxidant activity can be expressed as a dependence of the degree of discoloration on the concentration of the reference substance 6-hydroxy-2,5,7,8-tetramethylchroman-2-carboxylic acid (Trolox). Trolox is a water-soluble analogue of vitamin E with high antioxidant activity, commonly used as the reference substance. All reagents were purchased from Sigma-Aldrich (Sigma-Aldrich Co., St. Louis, MO, USA).

ABTS working solution was obtained by mixing equal volumes (1.0 mL) of the 14.0 mM ABTS stock solution with the 5.0 mM potassium persulfate stock solution in a 200 mL flask. The mixture was stored in the dark at room temperature for 16 h and then diluted with distilled water to a volume of 200 mL. Trolox standard solutions with final concentrations in the range of 0–10.0 μM were prepared by a series of dilutions of the 8.1 mM Trolox stock solution. Sample solutions were obtained by placing 0.10 g of the sample in a 10.0 mL flask and its dilution with distilled water to a volume of 10.0 mL. Solutions containing ZnO particles were centrifuged at 6000 rpm/4427 rcf for 2 min. A total of 50.0 μL of Trolox standard or the sample solution were added to 4.0 mL of the ABTS working solution in a 1 cm light-path polystyrene cuvette. Absorbance values were read at 734 nm before adding and 10 min after adding and mixing the content of the cuvette. For this purpose, a Thermo

Scientific Evolution 300 UV–Vis spectrophotometer (Thermo Fisher Scientific, Waltham, MA, USA) was used. Appropriate solvent blanks were run for the Trolox standards and the sample solutions. All determinations were carried out at least two times. The antioxidant activity results are given as TEAC values (mM Trolox).

The antimicrobial activity of the synthesized samples was tested against Gram-positive bacteria (*Staphylococcus aureus*—ATCC 6538), Gram-negative bacteria (*Pseudomonas aeruginosa*—ATCC 9027), and yeast (*Candida albicans*—ATCC 10231). An overnight broth culture of each strain was used to prepare inoculum. The suspensions of bacteria and yeast were adjusted to a density of 0.5 and 0.6 McFarland standard, which is 1.5×10^8 CFU/mL. Then, the cultures were diluted 100-fold into 10.0 mL of Mueller–Hinton Broth (Biomaxima) medium. The synthesized powders (BT1, BT2, BT3) were added to the respective cultures to a final concentration of 10 mg/mL. Cultures were incubated at 37 °C with shaking at 170 rpm and samples were collected at 2, 6, and 24 h. Samples were immediately diluted in normal saline (0.9%). The number of colony-forming units was determined using the Miles and Misra technique [44–46]. Briefly, TSA (trypticase soy agar) plates were divided into eight equal sectors, labeled with the dilution from 100 to 10^{-7}. In each sector, 3.0×10.0 µL of the appropriate dilution was dropped onto the agar surface. The plates were incubated at 37 °C for 24 h. The images of plates after a certain time of incubation were presented on the example of the BT1 sample and *S. aureus* bacteria (Figure S1). The CFU/mL and the percentage of the viability reduction was counted. The assay was done three times independently.

3. Results and Discussion

3.1. Black Tea Extract Spectral Analysis

As mentioned before, the chemical composition of a tea extract is very complex. It was reported that it consists of about four thousand bioactive compounds like polyphenols, phenols, phenolic acids, alkaloids, amino acids, carbohydrates, proteins, chlorophyll, and volatile organic compounds. The composition is not constant and depends on various factors, with the most important being the origin and age of the plant, and the method of preparation [47–49]. For these reasons, the exact composition always has to be confirmed.

The FTIR results indicated many peaks on the spectrum of black tea. These were associated with different functional groups: –OH (~3400 cm^{-1}), –CH (~2920 cm^{-1}), COOH (1697 cm^{-1}), COO$^-$ (1697, 1403 cm^{-1}), –CH$_2$ and CH$_3$ (1448, 1372 cm^{-1}), C–O–C (1231, 1030 cm^{-1}), –C–O (1145 cm^{-1}), aromatic ring (823, 758, 708 cm^{-1}), and –OH in phenols (612 cm^{-1}) (Figure S2). These attributions were made thanks to the literature data [47–49], however, due to the occurrence of similar functional groups in the mentioned compounds, it is very difficult to distinguish and name them only on the basis of these results.

To perform a detailed investigation of the chemical composition of the obtained black tea extract, LC-MS analyses were conducted. In total, 48 compounds were detected in both ion modes (Table S1). It was shown that the largest group of ingredients in black tea infusion were flavonoids, both aglycones and glycosides, from the flavan-3-ols (e.g., quercetin, kaempferol) and catechin (e.g., epicatechin, catechin, theaflavin) groups, constituting over two thirds of the identified compounds. Ten of the identified compounds were acids, mainly quinic acid, gallic acid, and *p*-coumaroylquinic acids. Moreover, the analysis also showed the presence of amino acids and an alkaloid (e.g., theanine and caffeine, respectively) [39,40].

3.2. Characterization of ZnO Particles

3.2.1. Chemical Structure

The FTIR measurements of the obtained samples confirmed a successful synthesis of ZnO particles, which was evident by the presence of Zn–O oscillation (~480 cm^{-1}). Additionally in the BT3 sample, the peaks characteristic for zinc hydroxide were observed (triplet ~2100, doublet ~1050, and 850 cm^{-1}), which were absent in the spectra of another measured materials. In addition, some oscillations connected with organic compounds of black tea extract were observed. They could be assigned to appropriate functional groups: –OH (~3400 cm^{-1}), C–H (~2900 cm^{-1}), COO$^-$ (~1576, 1406 cm^{-1}), C–OH (~1028 cm^{-1}), and aromatic ring (~880 cm^{-1}). The more black tea extract was used during ZnO synthesis, the more intensive these peaks were. This suggests that a larger amount of organic components was adsorbed on the zinc oxide surface (Figure 1a). This was also observed by a gradual color change within the samples from cream to brown (Figure 1b). Taking into account the spectroscopy analysis (FTIR, LC-MS) of the black tea extract and literature data [50–52], it could be concluded that the component adsorbed on the surface of ZnO was gallic acid. COO$^-$ groups were observed, so it could be supposed that zinc ions present on the ZnO surface can chemically interact with gallic acid. Taking into account the FTIR results and the literature data, this occurred most probably by complexing the metal ions with the hydroxyl groups of the acid [53,54] or carboxylic group. Additionally, in BT3, a new peak was observed at about 1480 cm^{-1}, which could be connected to C–O–C oscillations in esters (Figure 1a). It is supposed that gallic acid particles could interact not only with metal ions, but also between each other because of the autoxidation reaction. Other authors have suggested that as a result of this process, C–O (Figure 1c) or C–C (Figure 1d) bonded, ellagic acid (Figure 1e), or gallate-based polymers (Figure 1f) can occur [55–57]. The obtained FTIR results showed C–O–C bonding in the BT3 sample, which suggests that the C–O dimer, ellagic acid, or gellate-based polymer could be obtained.

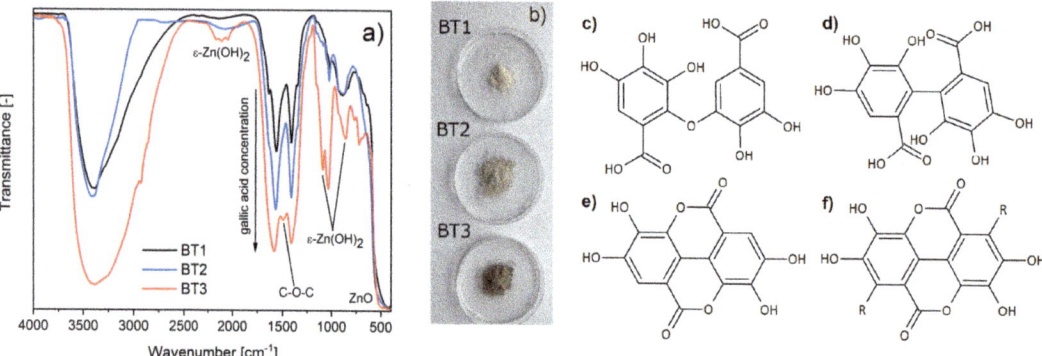

Figure 1. (**a**) FTIR spectra of the samples; (**b**) images of the samples; gallic acid autoxidation products: (**c**) C–O dimer, (**d**) C–C dimer, (**e**) ellagic acid, (**f**) gelate-based polymer.

3.2.2. Crystalline Structure

The diffractograms of the samples were different for each material. In the case of BT1 and BT2, only the wurtzite-type zinc oxide (ICDD 01-070-8070) was observed. In BT3, a hexagonal form of ZnO was also present, but the dominant one was wülfingite, which is a crystalline form of zinc hydroxide with orthorhombic unit cell (ε-Zn(OH)$_2$) (ICDD 04-012-2300). Additionally, a very small amount of zinc acetate (ZnAc) (ICDD 00-021-1467) fraction was indicated (Figure 2).

The authors obtained similar results when pectin was used as a stabilizing agent in the course of the synthesis of ZnO particles [6]. To understand the possible influence of black tea extract on zinc oxide crystallization, its mechanism has to be described. In the first step, the zinc ions were formed because of zinc acetate dissociation. After adding sodium hydroxide into the reaction mixture, the OH$^-$ anions were created, which could interact with zinc cations. As a result, amorphous zinc hydroxide will be obtained, which could further transform into crystalline ε-Zn(OH)$_2$ and then into ZnO.

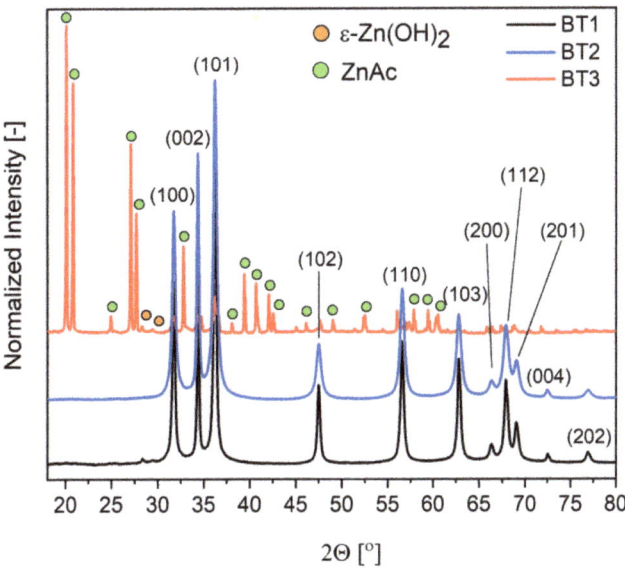

Figure 2. Diffractograms of the samples.

From the literature data, it is known that gallic acid has a great tendency to metal ion chelation [53,58,59]. For this reason, it could slow down the hydroxide precipitation process by temporarily blocking the cations. With the addition of hydroxide, the pH of the system gradually changes and the equilibrium state of the system shifts toward the formation of an amorphous and crystalline hydroxide phase. Thanks to that phenomenon, the crystallization process is controlled at this stage. Additionally, it is known that re-crystallization of ε-Zn(OH)$_2$ to ZnO occurs not by dissolution and liquid phase reactions, but by solid phase processes. The dehydration of the hydroxide begins inside the crystal and gradually progresses toward the outside. Therefore, the hydroxide residues are very often found on the surface of the final zinc oxide [60]. The obtained XRD results suggest that gallic acid can stabilize the hydroxide form and hinders its transformation into zinc oxide. This is evident by the fact that in samples (BT1, BT2) with the smaller amount of this organic component, only the wurtzite-type ZnO was observed on their surface. In the case of BT3, a very small amount of ZnO in the BT3 sample and very well crystallized ε-Zn(OH)$_2$ were present. These conclusions were also supported by FTIR results. Additionally, crystallite size (D) and microstrains (ε) of zinc oxide crystals were calculated using the Williamson–Hall equation [41]. The obtained results showed that in the case of the BT1 and BT3 samples, the D values decreased (23, 19 nm) and the ε values increased (0.04, 0.23) as a function of black tea concentration. In the BT3 sample, ZnO diffraction peaks were not intense enough to count these values as ε-Zn(OH)$_2$ was the dominant crystalline fraction. These observations could suggest that organic molecules adsorb on the particles' surface, which causes the disturbance in the decreasing size of the crystal structure of ZnO. Taking into account the literature data, most probably gallic acid interacts with the hydroxide group, which is blocking the dehydration process and stabilizes the ε-Zn(OH)$_2$ form [56]. The lack of a linear relationship between the amount of organic stabilizing agent and the amount of ε-Zn(OH)$_2$ suggests that there is a minimal concentration of gallic acid that is needed to block the transformation of crystalline hydroxide to oxide.

3.2.3. Morphology

Scanning electron microscopy indicated that the morphology of obtained ZnO particles depends on the amount of used black tea extract. In the case of the BT1 sample, the particles were in the form of nanoflakes, whose lengths and widths were around 100–550 and 21 nm, respectively (Figure 3a,b). BT2 particles had a nanocone-like shape (50–300 nm length and 30–175 nm width), which were agglomerates of smaller units (diameter ~14 nm) (Figure 3c,d). In the image of the BT3 sample, two kinds of structures were visible. One were small, quasi-spherical with a diameter of ~150 nm. The other structure had octahedral morphology and were much bigger with the side length around 3.5 μm (Figure 3e,f). It was supposed that they were separate fractions that may have a different material composition. The amount of octahedral structures were greater than the spherical ones. Based on the XRD and FTIR results, it could be concluded that small particles are made of hexagonal type ZnO crystals and octahedral are built from orthorhombic ε-Zn(OH)$_2$ [60–62].

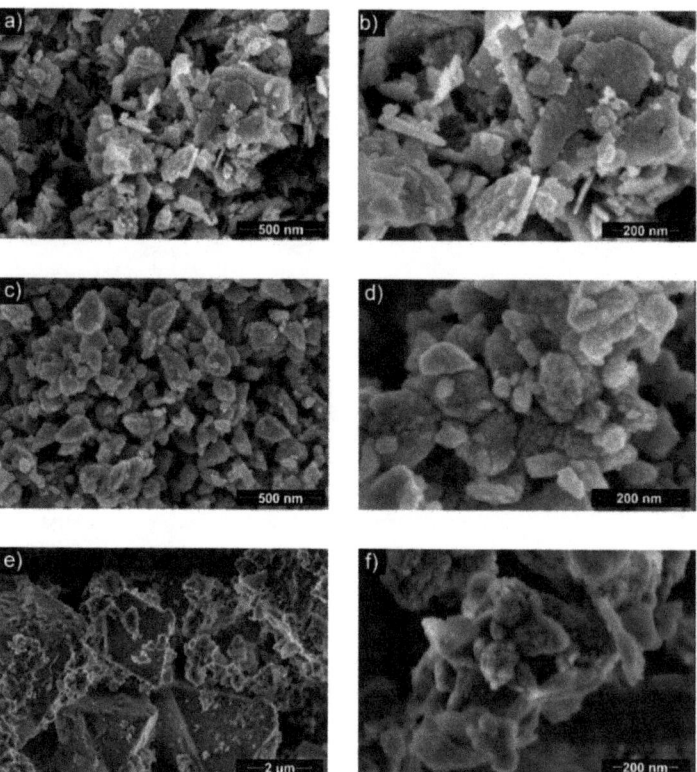

Figure 3. SEM images of the samples: (**a**,**b**) BT1, (**c**,**d**) BT2, (**e**,**f**) BT3.

Generally, it could be assumed that by increasing the amount of black tea extract, the particles change their shape and size starting from flat and big particles to more spherical and smaller. Additionally, in the BT3 sample, a fraction of a new material was obtained. Based on previous work by the authors [6], it was supposed that chemical components of the tea extract interact with ZnO crystallites. First, they adsorbed on the wurtzite polar surfaces (0001 and 000$\bar{1}$) and suppressed the growth along the c-axis [63]. By increasing the amount of organic compounds, they could start to adsorb on each side of the ZnO hexagonal unit cell, which inhibits its growth in every direction. Because the wülfingite fraction was observed in the BT3 sample, it could be concluded that the black tea extract may influence the process on each of its steps. This was reflected in an altered crystal growth and formation of various phases in the final product.

3.2.4. Thermal Analysis

Thermal stability of the samples obtained with the smallest and the biggest amount of the black tea extract was examined by thermogravimetric analysis. The results indicated that in the case of BT1, four mass losses were observed with the maximum degradation rates found at around 40, 160, 270, and 450 °C (Figure 4a). The observations for the BT3 sample were definitely different. Four degradation stages were also observed, however, the maxima were found at other temperatures: 80, 150, 195, and 330 °C (Figure 4b).

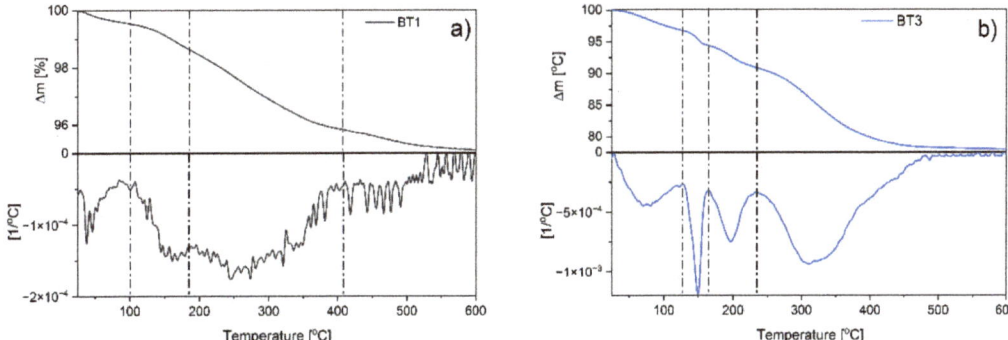

Figure 4. TG and DTG curves of: (**a**) BT1; (**b**) BT3 samples.

Based on FTIR, XRD, SEM analysis, and the authors' previous data [6], it could be supposed that moisture evaporation can be observed during the first step. Then, at around 150–160 °C, degradation of amorphous zinc hydroxide was observed. Further temperature increase caused ε-$Zn(OH)_2$ decomposition (~195 °C). Finally, the degradation of organic components occurs in different ways depending on the sample. In the case of BT1, the process was multi-stage and occurred at temperatures typical for gallic acid decomposition [53], which proves that the compound was adsorbed on the ZnO surface. In BT3, one stage was observed that took place at higher temperatures than BT1. This could confirm the conclusion postulated in FTIR studies about the interactions of gallic acid–gallic acid, which increase the thermal stability of the organic phase present on the ZnO surface.

Comparison of the values of individual weight losses were found to be significantly greater for the BT3 sample than for the BT1 at each degradation stage. The weight loss associated with moisture has increased from 0.46 to 3.23% and the loss connected with amorphous zinc hydroxide from 0.91 to 2.38%. ε-$Zn(OH)_2$ was present only in BT3 (3.48%). The gallic acid content was about 3.52% in BT1 and 13.45% in BT3 (Figure 4).

In summary, the TG results suggest that the more black tea extract was used, the more gallic acid molecules were adsorbed on the surface of the particles. This led to an increase in their tendency to adsorb moisture and block the transformation of both amorphous and crystalline zinc hydroxide to zinc oxide. Additionally, a large amount of gallic acid particles provokes their chemical interactions with each other, which was supported by the FTIR results.

In order to specify the interactions between gallic acid particles, the values of activation energy were determined as a function of materials conversion. In the case of BT1, the E_a value of amorphous $Zn(OH)_2$ was higher than in BT3. Supposedly, this fraction exhibits a stronger bond with the ZnO surface. In the BT3 sample, the degradation energy of ε-$Zn(OH)_2$ was also detected. In both cases, the decomposition of gallic acid is a two-step process, but the E_a values were higher in the BT3 sample. This was not noticeable on the thermogravimetric curves due to an overlap of processes at similar temperatures in the BT3 sample. These observations could indicate gallic acid–gallic acid interactions (Figure 5).

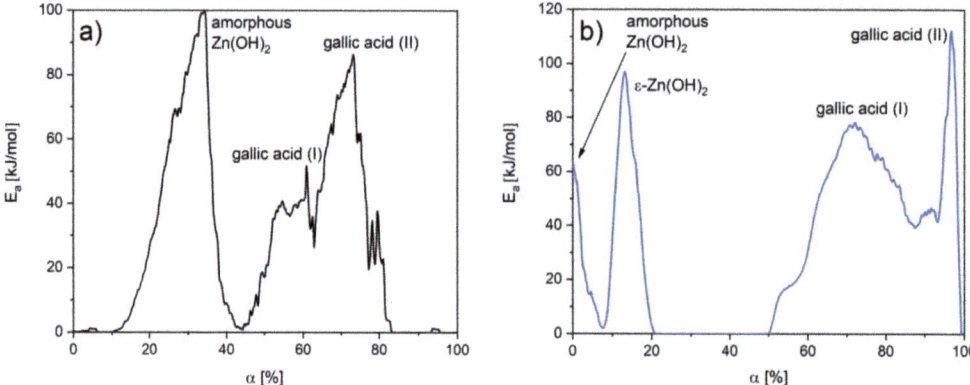

Figure 5. E_a changes as a function of conversion degree in the sample: (**a**) BT1, (**b**) BT3.

The spectral analyses of gas products evolving during decomposition were conducted to confirm the composition and the proposed degradation mechanism. Because of the largest amount of the additional fraction, the BT3 sample was tested. Both FTIR and QMS spectra showed that during the first three degradation steps, only water was detected. In the last step, only carbon dioxide was produced (Figure 6). This confirms the previous results obtained from other measurements and points to the proposed sample composition and its degradation mechanism.

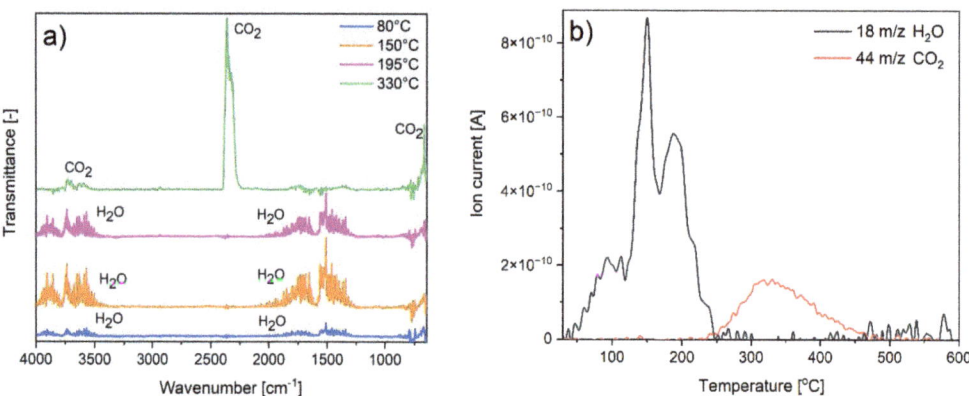

Figure 6. Spectra of evolving gaseous products: (**a**) FTIR; (**b**) QMS.

3.2.5. Antioxidative Properties

Black tea extract owes its antioxidant properties mainly to the presence of polyphenols [64]. Its concentration depends on many factors related to the processing of the leaves but also to the process of their infusion including the pH of the water used, the temperature, and the infusion time [65]. In this study, the antioxidant activity of black tea extract was calculated as 453.70 mM Trolox based on the ABTS assay. The obtained result was within the range of values found in the literature [66]. The obtained particles also showed antioxidant properties with values of 17.77, 43.60, and 63.32 mM Trolox for BT1, BT2, and BT3 samples, respectively. These results could be connected with the increasing concentration of the gallic acid on the ZnO surface in subsequent attempts, as demonstrated by the FTIR and TG measurements, which is most likely a result of the adsorption of gallic acid on the surface of particles. Based on the thermal analysis data, the gallic acid content was about

3.52% in BT1 and 13.45% in BT3. The difference of these concentrations between the BT3 and BT1 samples was about four times, which showed the same tendency as an increase in antioxidant activity and confirms the presented hypothesis.

As mentioned, many polyphenols exhibit antioxidant properties. This is connected with five main mechanisms: hydrogen atom transfer (HAT), single electron transfer (SET), sequential proton loss electron transfer (SPLET), sequential double proton loss electron transfer (SdPLET), or radical adduct formation (RAF). In all of them, the polyphenols play the role of a donor. The preferred process depends on the dissociation enthalpy of the hydroxyl group and the ionization potential of a measured polyphenol molecule [54]. The reaction environment also plays a crucial role. In aqua solutions, SPLET or SdPLET are dominant for free radical scavenging while in an anhydrous environment, HAT and RAF take place [67]. Gallic acid in its basic form is not the most active natural polyphenol. However, in the case of ionization of the carboxyl group, the enthalpy of hydroxyl groups is significantly reduced, which gives gallic acid the strongest antioxidant activity [54]. FTIR results showed that this form of the organic molecule was present in the measured particles. Additionally, it is known that in free radical scavenging, the most effective position of –OH group is the *para* position. The hydroxyl groups in *meta* positions stabilize formed radicals, which increase antioxidant capacity [68]. These two phenomena are most likely responsible for the high antioxidant activity of the obtained samples.

The differences between the activities of the particles could be connected not only with increasing gallic acid concentration between the samples, but also the opposite effect of ZnO. Similar conclusions were also demonstrated by other authors [69]. This oxide is inherently very non-stoichiometric, so its crystal structure may contain numerous defects such as interstitial oxygen or oxygen vacancies. Thanks to the presence of oxygen vacancies, depending on the environment, atmospheric oxygen or water molecules could be very easily adsorbed on the ZnO surface in the form of ions or radicals [8]. Due to this phenomenon, this material has oxidizing properties [15,70], which could lower the antioxidant capacity of the samples.

3.2.6. Antimicrobial Assay

The antimicrobial activity of the tested compounds was examined against two bacterial and one fungus strain. The reference strains of *Staphylococcus aureus* ATCC 6538–grape-like Gram-positive cluster, rod shaped Gram-negative *Pseudomonas aeruginosa* ATCC 9027, and fungus *Candida albicans* ATCC 10231 were used for the experiment. The antimicrobial activity was assessed by time-kill assays (Figure 7). The tested compounds showed diversified antimicrobial activity.

The Gram-positive strain was the most susceptible to all samples. The results showed that the reduction of *S. aureus* viability was increasing as a function of time. After 2 h, a very similar activity was observed in the case of BT2 and BT3, but the best effect was displayed by the BT1 sample. After 24 h of exposition, all materials exhibited a bactericidal effect (reduction of viability above 99%) (Figure 7a).

The obtained results for *P. aeruginosa* varied the most during the time of the experiment. At the beginning, the best activity was demonstrated by BT1 and BT2. The strongest antibacterial effect against *P. aeruginosa* was observed after 6 h post-inoculation and significantly decreased afterward. After 24 h, it was visible that the more gallic acid on the ZnO surface, the better the antibacterial activity was (Figure 7b).

The observed high antifungal activity decreased during the time of the experiment. The smallest decrease in the antifungal activity was observed for BT3. It was clearly visible that the reduction of viability decreased as a function of gallic acid concentration (Figure 7c).

Many aspects can cause the antimicrobial activity differences among the ZnO NPs. The most important seems to be the chemical composition, size, and morphology of the used active material and also the microbial structure [1,71].

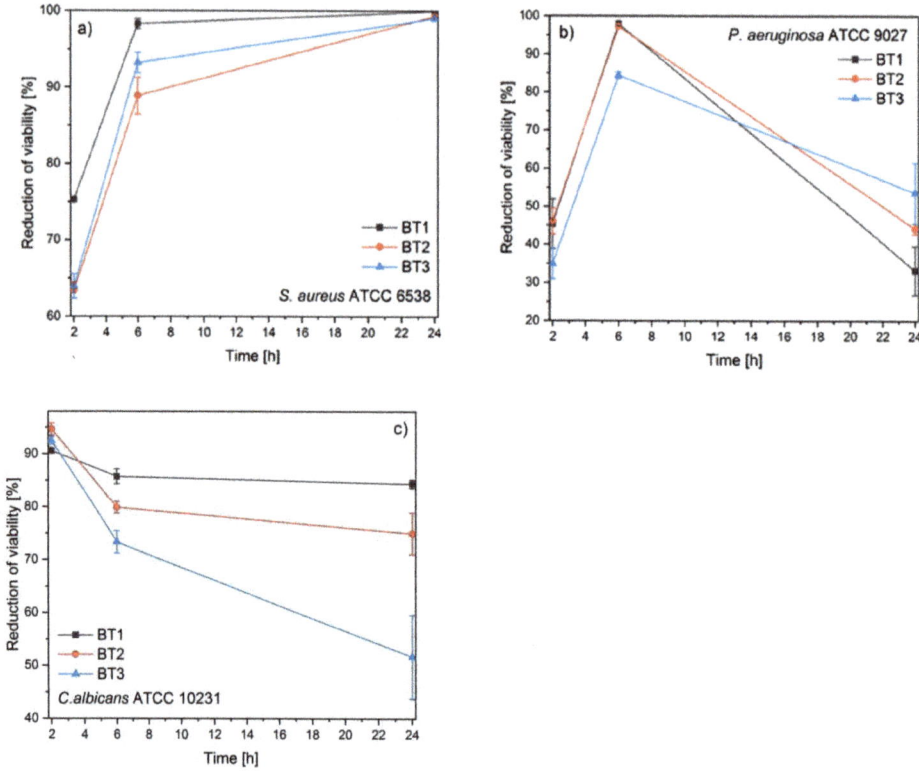

Figure 7. Antimicrobial activity of ZnO NPs against: (**a**) *S. aureus*, (**b**) *P. aeruginosa*; (**c**) *C. albicans*.

Zinc oxide is a very popular antibacterial and antifungal agent. Many authors have investigated the mechanism of its activity. It was postulated that the phenomenon is correlated with zinc ion release or free radical generation. The previous studies from the authors indicated that zinc hydroxide is responsible for ion formation and zinc oxide for ROS generation. The comparison of this observation with antimicrobial results clearly demonstrated that not ions, but ROS generation, is more responsible for ZnO biological activity [15]. Considering those, it could be supposed that the decrease in antimicrobial ability as a function of gallic acid concentration is connected with increasing zinc hydroxide content in the samples.

Additionally, the properties of gallic acid have to be considered. Because the black tea extract was used to obtain ZnO particles, its biological activity was determined. It was found that it did not reduce the growth of the tested microorganisms. However, in the literature data, it was demonstrated that pure gallic acid, due to its high tendency to ion and free radical binding, can interact with the microbial cell surface, which leads to a change in its hydrophobicity and charge. In the case of fungus, this organic molecule can interfere with 1,3-β-glucan and ergosterol synthase. All these processes cause a spill out of the cytoplasmic content [72].

To understand the antimicrobial activity of the measured samples, the ZnO–gallic acid interactions have to be taken into account. As mentioned before, the action of zinc oxide is mainly based on the generation of free radicals. Since gallic acid has strong antioxidant properties, the effect may be reduced. On the other hand, these components could show a synergistic effect thanks to the different action mechanisms.

In these studies, three microorganisms with significant differences in the cell wall structure were chosen.

Gram-positive bacteria have a thinner cell wall and are more sensitive to oxidative stress. The tested compounds showed a bactericidal effect against reference *S. aureus*, but the certain mechanisms of action are still unknown, although numerous studies pointing out the antibacterial effect of ZnO based compounds in the production of increased levels of ROS [73]. Since the activity of the tested samples is inversely proportional to the amount of gallic acid, it was suspected that it stabilizes the free radicals present on the ZnO surface by reducing their activity. Therefore, it takes longer to observe ROS interaction with the bacterial cell wall. In the presented studies, *S. aureus* exhibited the highest sensitivity to the obtained samples. These results are comparable with other research groups, which demonstrated that ZnO is more effective against Gram-positive strains [74]. Additionally, the bactericidal effect of the samples presented in this article was observed using a lower concentration of active material than that of the other authors [75] and its value is uncommon for particles of comparable sizes [71].

In contrast, *P. aeruginosa* is a Gram-negative strain that is known for its high resistance to antiseptic and other antimicrobial agents. This is probably due to its low outer membrane permeability. *Pseudomonas* has express specific channel proteins to nutrient incorporation and does not have general diffusion porins [76]. Despite the almost bacteriostatic activity after the first 6 h of the experiment, the persisted cells started to multiply and the antimicrobial activity decreased significantly. The observed decline in reduction of the viability was probably caused by *P. aeruginosa* cell wall structure and its properties. However, it has been shown that *P. aeruginosa* possesses antioxidant defenses including catalase production, which can increase its resistance to ROS produced during the activity of tested compounds [77,78]. After a long time of interaction between this Gram-negative strain and measured samples, their activity increased with gallic acid concentration. This could suggest that despite the start of building resistance against the action of free radicals, the used polyphenol may additionally connect with the cell wall and disrupt its proper functioning. Due to the highest resistance of Gram-negative strains toward antimicrobials, the obtained samples showed only an inhibitory effect on *P. aeruginosa* growth. The presented results were comparable with another author's study where the inhibitory effect was also observed using a similar concentration of ZnO [79].

Additionally, a fungistatic effect of the synthesized ZnO particles against *C. albicans* was observed. Based on the recent review, there were only a few studies on the antifungal activity of ZnO [71]. A similar analysis conducted by another author showed a comparable inhibitory effect after using a slightly smaller amount of the active ingredient [74]. This proved a high antimicrobial potential on the zinc oxide particles presented in this article. The different concentration used by other researchers needed to obtain a similar effect was likely due to the smaller particle size used in that test. Furthermore, *C. albicans*, as a representative of fungus, has a more complicated cell structure than bacteria. They are eukaryotic cells that have a uniquely composed two-layered cell wall structure. The main components are β-glucans, chitin, and mannoproteins [80], although ergosterol is one of the basal components of the *C. albicans* cell membranes responsible for its integrity [81]. One of the antifungal strategies described in the literature is to develop drugs that are binding to sterols that are present in the fungal cell membranes, leading to cell lysis [82]. A recent report indicated that gallic acid antifungal activity is associated with disturbing the ergosterol synthesis pathway, however, this needs further investigation for *C. albicans* species [54]. In this case, both the free radical production by zinc oxide and the interaction of gallic acid with the cell wall could generate the apoptosis process [83,84]. The obtained long-term results showed that fungi are much more susceptible to the generation of free radicals than the action of organic acid. Therefore, the capture of ROS by gallic acid weakens the biological activity of the tested samples.

4. Conclusions

The conducted studies demonstrated that a water black tea extract could be successfully used as the stabilizing agent during ZnO synthesis. The used natural extract consists of 48 organic ingredients. However, it was indicated that it was gallic acid that played a major role in the particle formation at many stages of the process.

First, it controls the crystallization process of ZnO by zinc ion chelation, which disturbs the hydroxide precipitation process by temporarily blocking the cations. Furthermore, the addition of NaOH to the reaction environment shifts the equilibrium state of the system toward the formation of an amorphous and crystalline hydroxide phase. Second, gallic acid molecules can be adsorbed on the particle's surface by interacting with their hydroxide group. Thanks to that, gallic acid controls the crystallite size, stabilizes the hydroxide form, and hinders its transformation into zinc oxide.

Analysis of the antioxidant properties indicated that they are proportional to the amount of the gallic acid molecules that were on the surface of ZnO particles, but are also correlated with oxidizing properties of ZnO.

In addition, in the case of the antimicrobial activity of obtained samples, the ZnO–gallic acid interactions seem to be crucial. On one hand, their presence may weaken each other's action, and on the other hand, act synergistically. This depends mainly on the type of the tested microorganisms and the duration of the action of the active agent.

Supplementary Materials: The following are available online at https://www.mdpi.com/article/10.3390/nano11071816/s1, Figure S1. Images of TSA plates after culturing and incubation with *S. aureus* ATCC 6538 at 37 °C for 24 h; Figure S2. FTIR spectrum of the black tea extract; Table S1: LC-MS results.

Author Contributions: M.F.-T. coordinated all parts of the project, performed the TG experiments, analyzed all results, and wrote the manuscript; A.D. synthesized the samples, conducted FTIR, and STA experiments, and edited the manuscript; B.P. analyzed the LC-MS results; J.C. (Joanna Czajkowska) and E.C. conducted antimicrobial analysis; R.J. performed XRD studies; M.W.-K. conducted antioxidative properties analysis; J.C. (Joanna Cybińska) supervised and edited the manuscript. All authors have read and agreed to the published version of the manuscript.

Funding: This work was financed by the Polish Ministry of Science and Higher Education (No. 205719/E 725/S/2018) from the research statutory grant for supporting the research potential in PORT in 2018.

Data Availability Statement: The data is included in the main text and the supplementary materials.

Conflicts of Interest: The authors declare no conflict of interest. The funders had no role in the design of the study; in the collection, analyses, or interpretation of data; in the writing of the manuscript, or in the decision to publish the results.

References

1. Tortella, G.; Rubilar, O.; Fincheira, P.; Pieretti, J.C.; Duran, P.; Lourenço, I.M.; Seabra, A.B. Bactericidal and Virucidal Activities of Biogenic Metal-Based Nanoparticles: Advances and Perspectives. *Antibiotics* **2021**, *10*, 783. [CrossRef] [PubMed]
2. Vidya, C.; Prabha, M.C.; Raj, M.A. Green mediated synthesis of zinc oxide nanoparticles for the photocatalytic degradation of Rose Bengal dye. *Environ. Nanotechnol. Monit. Manag.* **2016**, *6*, 134–138. [CrossRef]
3. Singh, R.; Hano, C.; Nath, G.; Sharma, B. Green Biosynthesis of Silver Nanoparticles Using Leaf Extract of *Carissa carandas* L. and Their Antioxidant and Antimicrobial Activity against Human Pathogenic Bacteria. *Biomolecules* **2021**, *11*, 299. [CrossRef]
4. Azizi, S.; Mohamad, R.; Bahadoran, A.; Bayat, S.; Rahim, R.A.; Ariff, A.; Saad, W.Z. Effect of annealing temperature on antimicrobial and structural properties of bio-synthesized zinc oxide nanoparticles using flower extract of *Anchusa italica*. *J. Photochem. Photobiol. B Biol.* **2016**, *161*, 441–449. [CrossRef]
5. Rasha, E.; Monerah, A.; Manal, A.; Rehab, A.; Mohammed, D.; Doaa, E. Biosynthesis of Zinc Oxide Nanoparticles from *Acacia nilotica* (L.) Extract to Overcome Carbapenem-Resistant Klebsiella pneumoniae. *Molecules* **2021**, *26*, 1919. [CrossRef]
6. Dmochowska, A.; Czajkowska, J.; Jędrzejewski, R.; Stawiński, W.; Migdał, P.; Fiedot-Toboła, M. Pectin based banana peel extract as a stabilizing agent in zinc oxide nanoparticles synthesis. *Int. J. Biol. Macromol.* **2020**, *165*, 1581–1592. [CrossRef]
7. Salayová, A.; Bedlovičová, Z.; Daneu, N.; Baláž, M.; Lukáčová Bujňáková, Z.; Balážová, Ľ.; Tkáčiková, Ľ. Green Synthesis of Silver Nanoparticles with Antibacterial Activity Using Various Medicinal Plant Extracts: Morphology and Antibacterial Efficacy. *Nanomaterials* **2021**, *11*, 1005. [CrossRef] [PubMed]

8. Fiedot-Toboła, M.; Suchorska-Woźniak, P.; Startek, K.; Rac-Rumijowska, O.; Szukiewicz, R.; Kwoka, M.; Teterycz, H. Correlation between Microstructure and Chemical Composition of Zinc Oxide Gas Sensor Layers and Their Gas-Sensitive Properties in Chlorine Atmosphere. *Sensors* **2020**, *20*, 6951. [CrossRef]
9. Abu Ali, T.; Pilz, J.; Schäffner, P.; Kratzer, M.; Teichert, C.; Stadlober, B.; Coclite, A.M. Piezoelectric Properties of Zinc Oxide Thin Films Grown by Plasma-Enhanced Atomic Layer Deposition. *Phys. Status Solidi Appl. Mater. Sci.* **2020**, *217*, 2000319. [CrossRef]
10. Rajamanickam, N.; Kanmani, S.S.; Jayakumar, K.; Ramachandran, K. On the possibility of ferromagnetism and improved dye-sensitized solar cells efficiency in TiO_2/ZnO core/shell nanostructures. *J. Photochem. Photobiol. A Chem.* **2019**, *378*, 192–200. [CrossRef]
11. Saharudin, K.; Sreekantan, S.; Basiron, N.; Khor, Y.; Harun, N.; Mydin, R.B.; Md Akil, H.; Seeni, A.; Vignesh, K. Bacteriostatic Activity of LLDPE Nanocomposite Embedded with Sol–Gel Synthesized TiO_2/ZnO Coupled Oxides at Various Ratios. *Polymers* **2018**, *10*, 878. [CrossRef]
12. Fiedot-Toboła, M.; Dmochowska, A.; Jędrzejewski, R.; Stawiński, W.; Kryszak, B.; Cybińska, J. Pectin-organophilized ZnO nanoparticles as sustainable fillers for high-density polyethylene composites. *Int. J. Biol. Macromol.* **2021**, *182*, 1832–1842. [CrossRef]
13. Abbas, M.; Buntinx, M.; Deferme, W.; Reddy, N.; Peeters, R. Oxygen Gas and UV Barrier Properties of Nano-ZnO-Coated PET and PHBHHx Materials Fabricated by Ultrasonic Spray-Coating Technique. *Nanomaterials* **2021**, *11*, 449. [CrossRef]
14. Mizielińska, M.; Nawrotek, P.; Stachurska, X.; Ordon, M.; Bartkowiak, A. Packaging Covered with Antiviral and Antibacterial Coatings Based on ZnO Nanoparticles Supplemented with Geraniol and Carvacrol. *Int. J. Mol. Sci.* **2021**, *22*, 1717. [CrossRef] [PubMed]
15. Fiedot, M.; Maliszewska, I.; Rac-Rumijowska, O.; Suchorska-Woźniak, P.; Lewińska, A.; Teterycz, H. The Relationship between the Mechanism of Zinc Oxide Crystallization and Its Antimicrobial Properties for the Surface Modification of Surgical Meshes. *Materials* **2017**, *10*, 353. [CrossRef]
16. Shateri-Khalilabad, M.; Yazdanshenas, M.E. Bifunctionalization of cotton textiles by ZnO nanostructures: Antimicrobial activity and ultraviolet protection. *Text. Res. J.* **2013**, *83*, 993–1004. [CrossRef]
17. Tang, G.Y.; Meng, X.; Gan, R.Y.; Zhao, C.N.; Liu, Q.; Feng, Y.B.; Li, S.; Wei, X.L.; Atanasov, A.G.; Corke, H.; et al. Health functions and related molecular mechanisms of tea components: An update review. *Int. J. Mol. Sci.* **2019**, *20*, 6196. [CrossRef] [PubMed]
18. Graham, H.N. Green tea composition, consumption, and polyphenol chemistry. *Prev. Med.* **1992**, *21*, 334–350. [CrossRef]
19. Islam, S.N.; Farooq, S.; Sehgal, A. Effect of consecutive steeping on antioxidant potential of green, oolong and black tea. *Int. J. Food Sci. Technol.* **2018**, *53*, 182–187. [CrossRef]
20. Tong, T.; Liu, Y.J.; Kang, J.; Zhang, C.M.; Kang, S.G. Antioxidant activity and main chemical components of a novel fermented tea. *Molecules* **2019**, *24*, 2917. [CrossRef] [PubMed]
21. Nadiah, N.I.; Cheng, L.H.; Azhar, M.E.; Karim, A.A.; Uthumporn, U.; Ruri, A.S. Determination of Phenolics and Antioxidant Properties in Tea and the Effects of Polyphenols on Alpha-Amylase Activity. *Pakistan J. Nutr.* **2015**, *14*, 808–817. [CrossRef]
22. Alqahtani, S.; Welton, K.; Gius, J.; Elmegerhi, S.; Kato, T. The Effect of Green and Black Tea Polyphenols on BRCA2 Deficient Chinese Hamster Cells by Synthetic Lethality through PARP Inhibition. *Int. J. Mol. Sci.* **2019**, *20*, 1274. [CrossRef] [PubMed]
23. Zuo, Y.; Chen, H.; Deng, Y. *Simultaneous Determination of Catechins, Caffeine and Gallic Acids in Green, Oolong, Black and pu-erh Teas Using HPLC with a Photodiode Array Detector*; Elsevier: Amsterdam, The Netherlands, 2002; Volume 57.
24. Sang, S.; Lambert, J.D.; Ho, C.T.; Yang, C.S. The chemistry and biotransformation of tea constituents. *Pharmacol. Res.* **2011**, *64*, 87–99. [CrossRef]
25. Xiao, J.B.; Jiang, H. A Review on the Structure-Function Relationship Aspect of Polysaccharides from Tea Materials. *Crit. Rev. Food Sci. Nutr.* **2015**, *55*, 930–938. [CrossRef] [PubMed]
26. Bi, W.; He, C.; Ma, Y.; Shen, J.; Zhang, L.H.; Peng, Y.; Xiao, P. Investigation of free amino acid, total phenolics, antioxidant activity and purine alkaloids to assess the health properties of non-Camellia tea. *Acta Pharm. Sin. B* **2016**, *6*, 170–181. [CrossRef]
27. Horanni, R.; Engelhardt, U.H. Determination of amino acids in white, green, black, oolong, pu-erh teas and tea products. *J. Food Compos. Anal.* **2013**, *31*, 94–100. [CrossRef]
28. Jiang, X.; Feng, K.; Yang, X. In vitro antifungal activity and mechanism of action of tea polyphenols and tea saponin against Rhizopus stolonifer. *J. Mol. Microbiol. Biotechnol.* **2015**, *25*, 269–276. [CrossRef] [PubMed]
29. Łuczaj, W.; Skrzydlewska, E. Antioxidative properties of black tea. *Prev. Med.* **2005**, *40*, 910–918. [CrossRef]
30. Lebaschi, S.; Hekmati, M.; Veisi, H. Green synthesis of palladium nanoparticles mediated by black tea leaves (*Camellia sinensis*) extract: Catalytic activity in the reduction of 4-nitrophenol and Suzuki-Miyaura coupling reaction under ligand-free conditions. *J. Colloid Interface Sci.* **2017**, *485*, 223–231. [CrossRef] [PubMed]
31. Çetinkaya, S.; Kütük, N. Green Synthesis of Iron Oxide Nanoparticles Using Black Tea Extract and Investigation of Its Properties. *Mater. Focus* **2018**, *7*, 316–320. [CrossRef]
32. Fardood, S.T.; Ramazani, A. Black Tea Extract Mediated Green Synthesis of Copper Oxide Nanoparticles. *J. Appl. Chem. Res.* **2018**, *12*, 8–15.
33. Asghar, M.A.; Zahir, E.; Shahid, S.M.; Khan, M.N.; Asghar, M.A.; Iqbal, J.; Walker, G. Iron, copper and silver nanoparticles: Green synthesis using green and black tea leaves extracts and evaluation of antibacterial, antifungal and aflatoxin B1 adsorption activity. *LWT Food Sci. Technol.* **2018**, *90*, 98–107. [CrossRef]

34. Banoee, M.; Mokhtari, N.; Sepahi, A.A.; Fesharaki, P.J.; Monsef-Esfahani, H.R.; Ehsanfar, Z.; Khoshayand, M.R.; Shahverdi, A.R. The green synthesis of gold nanoparticles using the ethanol extract of black tea and its tannin free fraction. *Iran. J. Mater. Sci. Eng.* **2010**, *7*, 48–53.
35. Yusoff, H.M.; Idris, N.H.; Fatin Hipul, N.; Fazila, N.; Yusoff, M.; Zafirah, N.; Izham, M.; Ul, I.; Bhat, H. Green Synthesis of Zinc Oxide Nanoparticles Using Black Tea Extract and its Potential as Anode Material in Sodium-Ion Batteries. *Malays. J. Chem.* **2020**, *22*, 43–51.
36. Fardood, S.T.; Ramazani, A.; Joo, S.W. Sol-gel Synthesis and Characterization of Zinc Oxide Nanoparticles Using Black Tea Extract. *J. Appl. Chem. Res.* **2017**, *11*, 8–17.
37. Nava, O.J.; Luque, P.A.; Gómez-Gutiérrez, C.M.; Vilchis-Nestor, A.R.; Castro-Beltrán, A.; Mota-González, M.L.; Olivas, A. Influence of Camellia sinensis extract on Zinc Oxide nanoparticle green synthesis. *J. Mol. Struct.* **2017**, *1134*, 121–125. [CrossRef]
38. Satheesha, K.S.; Bhat, R.; Tharani, M.; Rajeshkumar, S. In-Vitro Antibacterial Activity of Black Tea (*Camellia sinensis*) Mediated Zinc Oxide Nanoparticles Against Oral Pathogens. *Biosci. Biotechnol. Res. Commun.* **2020**, *13*. [CrossRef]
39. Araya-Farias, M.; Gaudreau, A.; Rozoy, E.; Bazinet, L. Rapid HPLC-MS method for the simultaneous determination of tea catechins and folates. *J. Agric. Food Chem.* **2014**, *62*, 4241–4250. [CrossRef]
40. Savic, I.; Nikolic, V.; Savic, I.; Nikolic, L.; Jovic, M.; Jovic, M. The qualitative analysis of the green tea extract using ESI-MS method. *Savrem. Tehnol.* **2014**, *3*, 30–37. [CrossRef]
41. Williamson, G.K.; Hall, W.H. X-ray line broadening from filed aluminium and wolfram. *Acta Metall.* **1953**, *1*, 22–31. [CrossRef]
42. Vyazovkin, S. Model-free kinetics: Staying free of multiplying entities without necessity. *J. Therm. Anal. Calorim.* **2006**, *83*, 45–51. [CrossRef]
43. Re, R.; Pellegrini, N.; Proteggente, A.; Pannala, A.; Yang, M.; Rice-Evans, C. Antioxidant activity applying an improved ABTS radical cation decolorization assay. *Free Radic. Biol. Med.* **1999**, *26*, 1231–1237. [CrossRef]
44. Miles, A.A.; Misra, S.S.; Irwin, J.O. The estimation of the bactericidal power of the blood. *Epidemiol. Infect.* **1938**, *38*, 732–749. [CrossRef]
45. De Matteis, V.; Cascione, M.; Toma, C.C.; Albanese, G.; De Giorgi, M.L.; Corsalini, M.; Rinaldi, R. Silver nanoparticles addition in poly(methyl methacrylate) dental matrix: Topographic and antimycotic studies. *Int. J. Mol. Sci.* **2019**, *20*, 4691. [CrossRef]
46. Thomas, P.; Sekhar, A.C.; Upreti, R.; Mujawar, M.M.; Pasha, S.S. Optimization of single plate-serial dilution spotting (SP-SDS) with sample anchoring as an assured method for bacterial and yeast cfu enumeration and single colony isolation from diverse samples. *Biotechnol. Rep.* **2015**, *8*, 45–55. [CrossRef] [PubMed]
47. Li, S.; Lo, C.Y.; Pan, M.H.; Lai, C.S.; Ho, C.T. Black tea: Chemical analysis and stability. *Food Funct.* **2013**, *4*, 10–18. [CrossRef]
48. Kc, Y.; Parajuli, A.; Khatri, B.B.; Shiwakoti, L.D. Phytochemicals and Quality of Green and Black Teas from Different Clones of Tea Plant. *J. Food Qual.* **2020**, *2020*, 8874271. [CrossRef]
49. Mukesh, R.; Namita, P.; Vijay, K.J. *Camellia Sinensis* (Green Tea): A Review. *Glob. J. Pharmacol.* **2012**, *6*, 52–59.
50. Naz, S.; Khaskheli, A.R.; Aljabour, A.; Kara, H.; Talpur, F.N.; Sherazi, S.T.H.; Khaskheli, A.A.; Jawaid, S. Synthesis of Highly Stable Cobalt Nanomaterial Using Gallic Acid and Its Application in Catalysis. *Adv. Chem.* **2014**, *2014*, 1–6. [CrossRef]
51. Boyatzis, S.C.; Velivasaki, G.; Malea, E. A study of the deterioration of aged parchment marked with laboratory iron gall inks using FTIR-ATR spectroscopy and micro hot table. *Herit. Sci.* **2016**, *4*, 1–17. [CrossRef]
52. Khaskheli, A.R.; Naz, S.; Ozul, F.; Aljabour, A.; Mahesar, S.A.; Patir, I.H.; Ersoz, M. Urchin-like cobalt nanostructures for catalytic degradation of nitro anilines. *Adv. Mater. Lett.* **2016**, *7*, 748–753. [CrossRef]
53. Masoud, M.S.; Hagagg, S.S.; Ali, A.E.; Nasr, N.M. Synthesis and spectroscopic characterization of gallic acid and some of its azo complexes. *J. Mol. Struct.* **2012**, *1014*, 17–25. [CrossRef]
54. Badhani, B.; Sharma, N.; Kakkar, R. Gallic acid: A versatile antioxidant with promising therapeutic and industrial applications. *RSC Adv.* **2015**, *5*, 27540–27557. [CrossRef]
55. Hotta, H.; Sakamoto, H.; Nagano, S.; Osakai, T.; Tsujino, Y. Unusually large numbers of electrons for the oxidation of polyphenolic antioxidants. *Biochim. Biophys. Acta Gen. Subj.* **2001**, *1526*, 159–167. [CrossRef]
56. Pant, A.F.; Özkasikci, D.; Fürtauer, S.; Reinelt, M. The Effect of Deprotonation on the Reaction Kinetics of an Oxygen Scavenger Based on Gallic Acid. *Front. Chem.* **2019**, *7*, 680. [CrossRef]
57. Tulyathan, V.; Boulton, R.B.; Singleton, V.L. Oxygen Uptake by Gallic Acid as a Model for Similar Reactions in Wines. *J. Agric. Food Chem.* **1989**, *37*, 844–849. [CrossRef]
58. Chan, S.; Kantham, S.; Rao, V.M.; Palanivelu, M.K.; Pham, H.L.; Shaw, P.N.; McGeary, R.P.; Ross, B.P. Metal chelation, radical scavenging and inhibition of Aβ42 fibrillation by food constituents in relation to Alzheimer's disease. *Food Chem.* **2016**, *199*, 14–24. [CrossRef]
59. Ruta, L.L.; Farcasanu, I.C. Interaction between polyphenolic antioxidants and *Saccharomyces cerevisiae* cells defective in heavy metal transport across the plasma membrane. *Biomolecules* **2020**, *10*, 1512. [CrossRef]
60. Nicholas, N.J.; Franks, G.V.; Ducker, W.A. The mechanism for hydrothermal growth of zinc oxide. *CrystEngComm* **2012**, *14*, 1232–1240. [CrossRef]
61. Wu, D.; Jiang, Y.; Liu, J.; Yuan, Y.; Wu, J.; Jiang, K.; Xue, D. Template Route to Chemically Engineering Cavities at Nanoscale: A Case Study of Zn(OH)$_2$ Template. *Nanoscale Res. Lett.* **2010**, *5*, 1779–1787. [CrossRef]
62. Top, A.; Çetinkaya, H. Zinc oxide and zinc hydroxide formation via aqueous precipitation: Effect of the preparation route and lysozyme addition. *Mater. Chem. Phys.* **2015**, *167*, 77–87. [CrossRef]

63. Iqbal, T.; Khan, M.A.; Mahmood, H. Facile synthesis of ZnO nanosheets: Structural, antibacterial and photocatalytic studies. *Mater. Lett.* **2018**, *224*, 59–63. [CrossRef]
64. Liu, S.; Huang, H. Assessments of antioxidant effect of black tea extract and its rationals by erythrocyte haemolysis assay, plasma oxidation assay and cellular antioxidant activity (CAA) assay. *J. Funct. Foods* **2015**, *18*, 1095–1105. [CrossRef]
65. Chang, M.Y.; Lin, Y.Y.; Chang, Y.C.; Huang, W.Y.; Lin, W.S.; Chen, C.Y.; Huang, S.L.; Lin, Y.S. Effects of infusion and storage on antioxidant activity and total phenolic content of black tea. *Appl. Sci.* **2020**, *10*, 2685. [CrossRef]
66. Almajano, M.P.; Carbó, R.; Jiménez, J.A.L.; Gordon, M.H. Antioxidant and antimicrobial activities of tea infusions. *Food Chem.* **2008**, *108*, 55–63. [CrossRef]
67. Medina, M.E.; Iuga, C.; Alvarez-Idaboy, J.R. Antioxidant activity of propyl gallate in aqueous and lipid media: A theoretical study. *Phys. Chem. Chem. Phys.* **2013**, *15*, 13137–13146. [CrossRef]
68. Wright, J.S.; Johnson, E.R.; DiLabio, G.A. Predicting the activity of phenolic antioxidants: Theoretical method, analysis of substituent effects, and application to major families of antioxidants. *J. Am. Chem. Soc.* **2001**, *123*, 1173–1183. [CrossRef]
69. Lee, J.; Choi, K.H.; Min, J.; Kim, H.J.; Jee, J.P.; Park, B.J. Functionalized ZnO nanoparticles with gallic acid for antioxidant and antibacterial activity against methicillin-resistant *S. aureus*. *Nanomaterials* **2017**, *7*, 365. [CrossRef]
70. Lakshmi Prasanna, V.; Vijayaraghavan, R. Insight into the Mechanism of Antibacterial Activity of ZnO: Surface Defects Mediated Reactive Oxygen Species Even in the Dark. *Langmuir* **2015**, *31*, 9155–9162. [CrossRef]
71. Gudkov, S.V.; Burmistrov, D.E.; Serov, D.A.; Rebezov, M.B.; Semenova, A.A.; Lisitsyn, A.B. A Mini Review of Antibacterial Properties of ZnO Nanoparticles. *Front. Phys.* **2021**, *9*, 49. [CrossRef]
72. Teodoro, G.R.; Ellepola, K.; Seneviratne, C.J.; Koga-Ito, C.Y. Potential use of phenolic acids as anti-*Candida* agents: A review. *Front. Microbiol.* **2015**, *6*, 1420. [CrossRef] [PubMed]
73. Raghupathi, K.R.; Koodali, R.T.; Manna, A.C. Size-dependent bacterial growth inhibition and mechanism of antibacterial activity of zinc oxide nanoparticles. *Langmuir* **2011**, *27*, 4020–4028. [CrossRef] [PubMed]
74. Azam, A.; Ahmed, A.S.; Oves, M.; Khan, M.S.; Habib, S.S.; Memic, A. Antimicrobial activity of metal oxide nanoparticles against Gram-positive and Gram-negative bacteria: A comparative study. *Int. J. Nanomed.* **2012**, *7*, 6003–6009. [CrossRef] [PubMed]
75. Dobrucka, R.; Dlugaszewska, J.; Kaczmarek, M. Cytotoxic and antimicrobial effects of biosynthesized ZnO nanoparticles using of *Chelidonium majus* extract. *Biomed. Microdev.* **2018**, *20*, 1–13. [CrossRef] [PubMed]
76. Chevalier, S.; Bouffartigues, E.; Bodilis, J.; Maillot, O.; Lesouhaitier, O.; Feuilloley, M.G.J.; Orange, N.; Dufour, A.; Cornelis, P. Structure, function and regulation of *Pseudomonas aeruginosa* porins. *FEMS Microbiol. Rev.* **2017**, *41*, 698–722. [CrossRef]
77. Ahmed, M.N.; Porse, A.; Abdelsamad, A.; Sommer, M.; Høiby, N.; Ciofu, O. Lack of the major multifunctional catalase kata in *pseudomonas aeruginosa* accelerates evolution of antibiotic resistance in ciprofloxacin-treated biofilms. *Antimicrob. Agents Chemother.* **2019**, *63*, e00766-19. [CrossRef]
78. Elkins, J.G.; Hassett, D.J.; Stewart, P.S.; Schweizer, H.P.; McDermott, T.R. Protective role of catalase in *Pseudomonas aeruginosa* biofilm resistance to hydrogen peroxide. *Appl. Environ. Microbiol.* **1999**, *65*, 4594–4600. [CrossRef]
79. Saleh, M.M.; Refa't A, S.; Latif, H.K.A.; Abbas, H.A.; Askoura, M. Zinc oxide nanoparticles inhibits quorum sensing and virulence in *Pseudomonas aeruginosa*. *Afr. Health Sci.* **2019**, *19*, 2043–2055. [CrossRef]
80. Garcia-Rubio, R.; de Oliveira, H.C.; Rivera, J.; Trevijano-Contador, N. The Fungal Cell Wall: *Candida*, *Cryptococcus*, and *Aspergillus* Species. *Front. Microbiol.* **2020**, *10*, 2993. [CrossRef]
81. Lv, Q.Z.; Yan, L.; Jiang, Y.Y. The synthesis, regulation, and functions of sterols in *Candida albicans*: Well-known but still lots to learn. *Virulence* **2016**, *7*, 649–659. [CrossRef]
82. Richter, R.K.; Mickus, D.E.; Rychnovsky, S.D.; Molinski, T.F. Differential modulation of the antifungal activity of amphotericin B by natural and ent-cholesterol. *Bioorg. Med. Chem. Lett.* **2004**, *14*, 115–118. [CrossRef] [PubMed]
83. Altaf, R.; Asmawi, M.Z.B.; Dewa, A.; Sadikun, A.; Umar, M.I. Phytochemistry and medicinal properties of *Phaleria macrocarpa* (Scheff.) Boerl. extracts. *Pharmacogn. Rev.* **2013**, *7*, 73–80. [CrossRef] [PubMed]
84. Zhu, S.; Gong, L.; Li, Y.; Xu, H.; Gu, Z.; Zhao, Y. Safety Assessment of Nanomaterials to Eyes: An Important but Neglected Issue. *Adv. Sci.* **2019**, *6*, 1802289. [CrossRef] [PubMed]

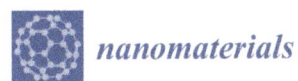

Article

Green Synthesis of Silver Nanoparticles Using *Diospyros malabarica* Fruit Extract and Assessments of Their Antimicrobial, Anticancer and Catalytic Reduction of 4-Nitrophenol (4-NP)

Kaushik Kumar Bharadwaj [1,†], Bijuli Rabha [1,†], Siddhartha Pati [2,3,†], Bhabesh Kumar Choudhury [4], Tanmay Sarkar [5,6], Sonit Kumar Gogoi [4], Nayanjyoti Kakati [1], Debabrat Baishya [1,*], Zulhisyam Abdul Kari [7,*] and Hisham Atan Edinur [8,*]

1. Department of Bioengineering and Technology, Gauhati University Institute of Science and Technology, Guwahati 781014, Assam, India; kkbhrdwj01@gmail.com (K.K.B.); bijulipep@gmail.com (B.R.); nayanjyotikakati0@gmail.com (N.K.)
2. SIAN Institute, Association for Biodiversity Conservation and Research (ABC), Balasore 756001, Odisha, India; patisiddhartha@gmail.com
3. Centre of Excellence, Khallikote University, Berhampur, Ganjam 761008, Odisha, India
4. Department of Chemistry, Gauhati University, Guwahati 781014, Assam, India; bkcsat@gmail.com (B.K.C.); skgogoi@gauhati.ac.in (S.K.G.)
5. Malda Polytechnic, West Bengal State Council of Technical Education, Government of West Bengal, Malda 732102, West Bengal, India; tanmays468@gmail.com
6. Department of Food Technology and Biochemical Engineering, Jadavpur University, Kolkata 700032, West Bengal, India
7. Faculty of Agro Based Industry, Universiti Malaysia Kelantan, Jeli 17600, Kelantan, Malaysia
8. School of Health Sciences, Health Campus, Universiti Sains Malaysia, Kubang Kerian 16150, Kelantan, Malaysia
* Correspondence: drdbaishya@gmail.com (D.B.); zulhisyam.a@umk.edu.my (Z.A.K.); edinur@usm.my (H.A.E.)
† These authors contributed equally to this work.

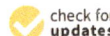

Citation: Bharadwaj, K.K.; Rabha, B.; Pati, S.; Choudhury, B.K.; Sarkar, T.; Gogoi, S.K.; Kakati, N.; Baishya, D.; Kari, Z.A.; Edinur, H.A. Green Synthesis of Silver Nanoparticles Using *Diospyros malabarica* Fruit Extract and Assessments of Their Antimicrobial, Anticancer and Catalytic Reduction of 4-Nitrophenol (4-NP). *Nanomaterials* **2021**, *11*, 1999. https://doi.org/10.3390/nano11081999

Academic Editor: Giovanni Benelli

Received: 30 June 2021
Accepted: 30 July 2021
Published: 4 August 2021

Publisher's Note: MDPI stays neutral with regard to jurisdictional claims in published maps and institutional affiliations.

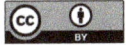

Copyright: © 2021 by the authors. Licensee MDPI, Basel, Switzerland. This article is an open access article distributed under the terms and conditions of the Creative Commons Attribution (CC BY) license (https://creativecommons.org/licenses/by/4.0/).

Abstract: The green synthesis of silver nanoparticles (AgNPs) has currently been gaining wide applications in the medical field of nanomedicine. Green synthesis is one of the most effective procedures for the production of AgNPs. The *Diospyros malabarica* tree grown throughout India has been reported to have antioxidant and various therapeutic applications. In the context of this, we have investigated the fruit of *Diospyros malabarica* for the potential of forming AgNPs and analyzed its antibacterial and anticancer activity. We have developed a rapid, single-step, cost-effective and eco-friendly method for the synthesis of AgNPs using *Diospyros malabarica* aqueous fruit extract at room temperature. The AgNPs began to form just after the reaction was initiated. The formation and characterization of AgNPs were confirmed by UV-Vis spectrophotometry, XRD, FTIR, DLS, Zeta potential, FESEM, EDX, TEM and photoluminescence (PL) methods. The average size of AgNPs, in accordance with TEM results, was found to be 17.4 nm. The antibacterial activity of the silver nanoparticles against pathogenic microorganism strains of *Staphylococcus aureus* and *Escherichia coli* was confirmed by the well diffusion method and was found to inhibit the growth of the bacteria with an average zone of inhibition size of (8.4 ± 0.3 mm and 12.1 ± 0.5 mm) and (6.1 ± 0.7 mm and 13.1 ± 0.5 mm) at 500 and 1000 µg/mL concentrations of AgNPs, respectively. The anticancer effect of the AgNPs was confirmed by MTT assay using the U87-MG (human primary glioblastoma) cell line. The IC_{50} value was found to be 58.63 ± 5.74 µg/mL. The results showed that green synthesized AgNPs exhibited significant antimicrobial and anticancer potency. In addition, nitrophenols, which are regarded as priority pollutants by the United States Environmental Protection Agency (USEPA), can also be catalytically reduced to less toxic aminophenols by utilizing synthesized AgNPs. As a model reaction, AgNPs are employed as a catalyst in the reduction of 4-nitrophenol to 4-aminophenol, which is an intermediate for numerous analgesics and antipyretic drugs. Thus, the study is expected to help immensely in the pharmaceutical industries in developing antimicrobial drugs and/or as an anticancer drug, as well as in the cosmetic and food industries.

Keywords: silver nanoparticles; *Diospyros malabarica*; antibacterial; anticancer; catalyst; 4-nitrophenol

1. Introduction

Nowadays, nanotechnology is a rapidly developing field and has a wide range of applications in biomedicine, drug delivery, bioimaging, bio-sensing devices, optoelectronics, catalysis and also in environmental protection due to the exemplary properties, such as biocompatibility, high productivity, rapid production and cost-effectiveness [1–5]. Among nanomaterials, metal nanoparticles, such as silver, copper, zinc, gold, titanium and magnesium, have been gaining immense magnitude for their applications and play a major role in this field [6–9]. In recent years, silver nanoparticles (AgNPs) have created attention among researchers because of their important applications in biomedicine, agriculture, food industry, catalytic, biosensors, optoelectronics and optics [10]. Several physical and chemical methods have been widely employed for the synthesis of AgNPs, such as sonochemical, microwave, γ-rays, hydrothermal, wet chemical, laser ablation and sol-gel, but these methods have some disadvantages, such as their use of high beam energy, hazardous toxic wastes, require high capital costs and production of large amounts of toxic byproducts that cause environmental contamination [11–13]. Hence, there is a need to develop eco-friendly techniques without using toxic chemicals to overcome these limitations. Green synthesis of AgNPs is rapidly increasing due to its enhanced stability, nontoxicity, inexpensive, eco-friendly, simple and rapid method of preparation approaches, which are substitutes to hazardous physical and chemical methods. Green synthesized AgNPs from plants are being successfully employed in various pharmaceutical and biomedical fields, such as antimicrobial, antibiofilm, antifungal, anticancer, anti-angiogenic therapy, anti-inflammatory, antioxidant, antiviral, drug delivery systems, gene therapy, bioimaging and wound healing [14–23].

Among different organic pollutants in water, 4-nitrophenol (4-NP) is a toxic and harmful agent more often found in industrial and agricultural raw materials that pose negative impacts on the environment and human health [24,25]. It is important to remove such pollutants from water before any use, including domestic and industrial use. In the current study, it is observed that the researcher is devoted to converting the organic pollutants to less hazardous products in the aqueous medium. The 4-aminophenol (4-AP), a reduced product of 4-NP, has extensive use in the production of analgesic and antipyretic drugs. The 4-AP is also used as an anti-corrosion agent, hair dyeing agent or photographic developer. In general, the reduction of 4-NP to 4-AP is catalyzed by an iron/acid catalyst that poses major environmental impacts [26]. The use of corrosive acids in large-scale production can be achieved by using metal nanoparticles as a catalyst along with sodium borohydride ($NaBH_4$). This method is found to be environmentally friendly. Despite thermal and electrical conduction, silver nanoparticles bear efficient catalytic properties. Silver nanoparticles can be synthesized using chemical, radiation, photochemical, Langmuir–Blodgettmethods, etc. [23]. However, green synthesis of silver nanostructures has received wide acceptance, as it possesses little hazard to the environment and human health [27]. Silver nanoparticles proved to have a unique increased ability to inhibit bacterial growth with no or negligible side effects when compared to antibiotics [28]. Cyclophanes synthesized AgNPs have shown wide applications in creating electrochemical and colorimetric sensors for the determination of heavy metal cations (Cu^{2+}, Fe^{3+}, Hg^{2+}, Cd^{2+}, Pb^{2+}) anions ($H_2PO_4^-$, I^-), amino acids, polycyclic aromatic hydrocarbons and pesticides [29].

For the green synthesis of metal nanoparticles, natural products, such as extracts from various plants or parts of plants (leaves, fruits, flower, bark, peel, seed, root, latex) have received the most attention due to their growing success [30–33]. The plant extracts contain various phytocompounds that act as capping, as well as reducing agents for the synthesis of nanoparticles [34]. The antioxidant polyphenols and flavonoids are the major phytocompounds, mainly responsible for the formation of AgNPs by the reduction of silver ions into silver metal (Ag⁺ to Ag) and also act as a capping agent that stabilizes the size of the formed nanoparticles and shaped during the synthesis of nanoparticles. These phytocompounds also have a tendency to absorb on the surface of nanoparticles [35,36]. In the green synthesis of nanoparticles using plant extracts, nature, the concentration of the plant extract, metal salt, pH, temperature and incubation time during reaction affect the rate, production amount and properties of the formed nanoparticles [37]. Different plant extracts including *Azadirachta indica*, *Anthemis atropatana*, *Benincasa hispida*, *Bauhinia variegata*, *Catharanthus roseus*, *Caesalpinia pulcherrima*, *Coriandrum sativum*, *Melissa officinalis*, *Pedalium murex*, *Prosopis juliflora*, *Parkia speciosa*, *Stigmaphyllo novatum*, *Cotyledon orbiculata*, *Diospyros lotus* and Andean blackberry leaf have been successfully reported for the biosynthesis of AgNPs [15,16,32,38–48].

Diospyros malabarica, a species of flowering tree belonging to the family Ebenaceae, grows throughout India and other tropical regions of the world. The fruit of the *Diospyros malabarica* tree are round and yellow when ripe during the month of July and August. Additionally, *D. malabarica* has been reported to have various therapeutic applications [49]. This tree was also reported to be used in traditional medicinal practices in various diseases. Various bioactive compounds, such as gallic acid, flavonoid, anthocyanin, saponin, alkaloid, vitamin C, tannins, triterpenes, sitosterol and betulinic acid, are being reported to be present, which are mainly responsible for their antioxidant, antiprotozoal, antihelminthic, antiviral and anticancer activity [49,50]. We hypothesized that these phytoconstituents could be applied in the green synthesis of AgNPs. Considering the importance of the green synthesis of silver nanoparticles using different plants and the various medicinal properties of the *Diospyros malabarica* plant, it has been indicative for delving into the present study. This study focused on the green synthesis of AgNPs using *Diospyros malabarica* aqueous fruit extract as a reducing and stabilizing agent. The formed AgNPs were characterized by using UV-Visible spectroscopy, TEM, FESEM, EDX, XRD, FT-IR, DLS, PDI, zeta potential and photoluminescence (PL) properties. Furthermore, the antimicrobial activities of synthesized AgNPs were evaluated against human pathogenic microorganisms *Escherichia coli* and *Staphylococcus aureus*, as well as anticancer activity investigated on U87-MG (human primary glioblastoma) cell lines. The catalytic activity for the reduction of 4-nitrophenol was also tested for produced AgNPs.

2. Materials and Methods

2.1. Materials

Analytical grade silver nitrate (AgNO$_3$) was procured from Sigma-Aldrich. Muller Hilton agar (MHA) for microbiology experiments was procured from HIMEDIA Laboratories (Mumbai, India). The bacterial pathogens *Escherichia coli* and *Staphylococcus aureus* used for the antimicrobial susceptibility evaluation were purchased from the Microbial Type Culture Collection (MTCC, Chandigarh, India). *Diospyros malabarica* fruit was freshly collected from the Morigaon district of Assam, India. Dulbecco's modified Eagle's medium (DMEM), fetal bovine serum (FBS) and MTT reagent (3-(4,5-dimethylthiazol-2-yl)-2,5-diphenyl tetrazolium bromide dye) was purchased from Sigma-Aldrich. The U87-MG (human primary glioblastoma) cell lines were obtained from the National Centre for Cell Science (NCCS), Pune, India.

2.2. Diospyros Malabarica (Aqueous) Fruit Extracts Preparation

The fruit of *Diospyros malabarica* was washed with tap water followed by distilled water until all the impurities were removed. Then, 20 g of fruit was weighed and immersed in 100 mL of double-distilled water (ddH$_2$O) in an Erlenmeyer flask, were kept on a heated plate (60 °C) and allowed to boil for 15 min. The fruit extract was filtered by using Whatman filter paper no. 1. Pellets were removed, and the supernatant was collected in another tube. The filtrate (supernatant) was further kept refrigerated at 4 °C for the synthesis of AgNPs.

2.3. Biosynthesis of AgNPs

For the green synthesis of AgNPs, silver nitrate AgNO$_3$ (99.98%) reagent grade was used as a precursor. A total of 1 mM AgNO$_3$ solution was prepared in ddH$_2$O from a stock solution of 1 M AgNO$_3$. Filtered aqueous fruit extract of *Diospyros malabarica* was mixed with this 1 mM AgNO$_3$ solution in a 1:9 mL ratio in a conical flask and kept in the dark at 24 °C for incubation for 1 h. After the passage of time, the synthesis progress (reduction of Ag$^+$ ions) was monitored by visual observation of change in color from light brown to dark brown. The color change indicates nanoparticle synthesis. Then, the green synthesized AgNPs were collected by centrifugation of 10,000 rpm for 15 min, and the precipitate was collected, washed with deionized water, dried and stored at room temperature. A schematic representation of AgNPs synthesis and its applications used in this study is depicted in Figure 1.

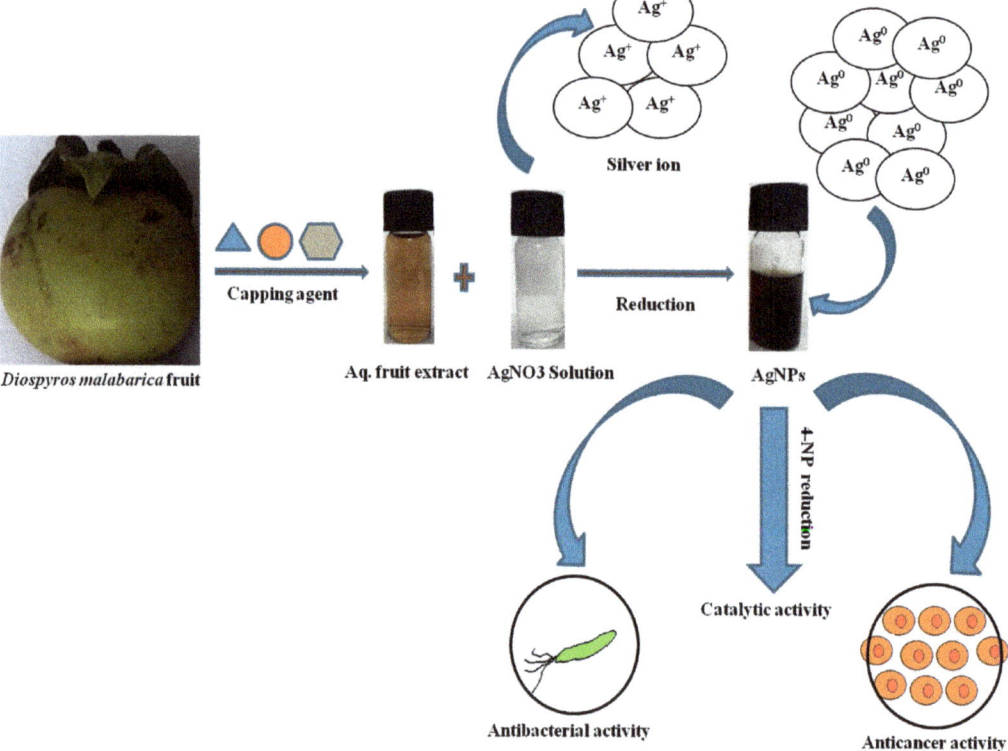

Figure 1. Schematic representation of the green synthesis of silver nanoparticles (AgNPs) and their applications.

2.4. Characterization of AgNPs

2.4.1. UV-Visible Spectroscopic Profile of Synthesized AgNPs

UV-Vis spectroscopy is the most important, simplest and most basic technique to confirm the formation of synthesized nanoparticles. UV-Vis spectra were recorded in the range between 300 and 700 nm using Cary 60 UV-Vis (Agilent Technologies, Santa Clara, CA, USA). In order to check the formation and stability of AgNPs, their SPR bands were recorded at different time intervals (0.5, 1, 1.5, 2, 2.5 and 4 h, respectively) during the green synthesis process. Double distilled water (ddH$_2$O) was used as a blank to adjust the baseline.

2.4.2. Stability of the Synthesized AgNPs

The stability of the green synthesized AgNPs from aqueous fruit extract of *Diospyros malabarica* in aqueous dispersions was determined by UV-Vis spectroscopy. The synthesized AgNPs were deliberately stored in a dark environment at ~30 °C. Afterward, the changes in the samples were monitored by UV-Vis spectra at 1 day and 60 days [51,52].

2.4.3. Transmission Electron Microscopy (TEM)

TEM was applied to depict the morphology, size and particle size distribution of the green synthesized AgNPs. The images were taken by JEOL 2100 Electron Microscope (JEOL, Peabody, MA, USA). For TEM analysis, a single drop (10 µL) of AgNPs suspension was placed on the carbon-coated copper grid, dried for 2 h at room temperature (24 °C) and loaded into the specimen holder before performing analysis at 120 kV accelerating voltage.

2.4.4. Field Emission Scanning Electron Microscope (FESEM) and Energy-Dispersive X-ray Spectroscopy (EDX)

To study the cell surface topography and characterize the elemental composition of synthesized AgNPs, FESEM combined with EDX were analyzed by using Sigma 300 (Carl Zeiss, Germany), operated at a 20 KV. A small amount of AgNPs (10 µL) was drop-cast on a clean coverslip and dried. The samples were then sputtered with gold and observed under a FESEM and EDX [53].

2.4.5. PolydispersityIndex (PDI), Particle Size (DLS) and Zeta Potential (ζ)

The quantification of size (DLS), polydispersity index (PDI) and ζ-potential of the synthesized AgNPs was carried out using a Zetasizer Nano ZS90 (Malvern, UK). The PDI determines the spread of the particle size distribution. DLS analysis determines the hydrodynamic radius by approximating the particle size of the synthesized AgNPs. ζ-potential measures the surface charge of the synthesized AgNPs nanoparticles.

2.4.6. X-ray Diffraction (XRD)

XRD measurement was carried out by Phillips X'Pert Pro powder X-ray diffractometer (XRD) (PANalytical, Almelo, The Netherlands) with a copper target (CuKα1, λ = 1.54056 Å). It was operated with a nickel filter at a voltage of 40 kV and a current of 45 mA [54].

2.4.7. Fourier Transform Infrared (FTIR)

To study the functional group present on the synthesized AgNPs surface, FTIR analysis was performed by using an FTIR spectrophotometer (Perkin Elmer spectrum 100 FTIR, 710 Bridgeport, CT, USA). The FT-IR spectra were scanned with wave numbers ranging between 4000 and 400 cm^{-1} at a resolution of 4 cm^{-1} in the transmittance mode [3].

2.4.8. Photoluminescence (PL)

The PL spectra of biosynthesized silver nanoparticles were recorded by using the spectrofluorometer (Jasco, Oklahoma City, OK, USA, FP-8300).

2.4.9. Antibacterial Activity of AgNPs

The antibacterial activities of the silver nanoparticles (AgNPs) were assessed against strains of clinical pathogenic microorganisms, *Escherichia coli* (*E. coli*) and *Staphylococcus aureus* (*S. aureus*), by using the agar well diffusion method [55]. Sterile and solidified Muller Hinton agar (20 mL) plates were swabbed with the microbes. Four wells were bored on each plate using a sterile well cutter, and all the experimental samples were given in triplicate in each plate. The wells were loaded with *Diospyros malabarica* aqueous fruit extracts (1000 µg/mL, 50 µL), synthesized AgNPs (500 and 1000 µg/mL, 50 µL) and double-distilled water (ddH$_2$O) as the negative control (50 µL), respectively. Three antibiotics (Streptomycin 10 µg, Tetracycline 30 µg and Chloramphenicol 30 µg) were loaded and tested against *E. coli* and *S. aureus* in each plate as the positive control. After

24 h of incubation at 37 °C, the zone of inhibition was measured in mm for bacterial strains. The experiments were repeated thrice, and the diameter of the zone of inhibition was expressed as mean ± standard deviation (SD).

2.4.10. Assessment of Cytotoxicity in U87-MG Cells

The human cancer cell lines U87-MG (human primary glioblastoma) were grown as a monolayer in DMEM, supplemented with heat-inactivated 10% FBS and 1% antibiotic. The cell lines were maintained and grown at 37 °C with a humidified atmosphere containing 5% CO_2 and 95% air. Both the cancerous cell lines (1×10^4 cells/well) were seeded in a 96-well microtiter plate and incubated at 37 °C for 24 h. After incubation, various concentrations (µg/mL) of synthesized AgNPs were treated in triplicates and incubated at 37 °C for 48 h. Then, the cytotoxicity was checked by MTT cytotoxicity assay. The media of 96-well plates were discarded, followed by the addition of 100 µL of MTT dye (5 mg/mL in phosphate buffer saline (PBS; pH 7.4)) in each well and incubated at 37 °C for 4 h. After incubation, MTT was removed, and dimethyl sulfoxide (DMSO; 100 µL) was added to dissolve the formazan crystals formed due to reduced MTT, and the absorbance was recorded. A microplate reader SYNERGY-H1 (Biotek) was used to estimate the amount of reduced MTT by measuring the optical density (OD) at 570 nm with a reference filter of 655 nm [39]. The IC_{50} value was calculated by using the following equation:

$$\text{Cell viability (\%)} = \frac{\text{Absorbance of sample}}{\text{Absorbace of control}} \times 100$$

Cell Morphology of AgNPs Treated U87-MG Cells

The morphology of the U87-MG cells after the treatment of synthesized AgNPs was studied under an inverted microscope. A total of 1×10^4 cells were seeded in 96-well plates in DMEM along with 10% FBS and incubated for 24 h at 37 °C in a CO_2 incubator. After incubation, U87-MG cells were again incubated for 24 h with the treatment of 1 mg/mL of synthesized AgNPs as treated and without AgNPs as untreated. The comparative effect on the morphology of the U87-MG cells of both treated and untreated was evaluated.

2.4.11. Live/Dead Assay

A live/dead assay was performed for the qualitative assessment of cell viability after treatment of synthesized AgNPs. The U87-MG cell lines at a density of 2×10^4 cells were seeded in 96-well plates for 24 h. After incubation, cells are treated with AgNPs concentrations of 1 mg/mL. A blank (without treatment) was kept for control. After incubation, the cells were washed with PBS (pH 7.4) and stained with propidium iodide (PI) and thiazole orange (TO). The plates were then incubated for 45 min and observed using a confocal laser scanning microscope (CLSM) (TCS SP8, Leica, Germany).

2.4.12. Catalytic Activity Test for Reduction of 4-Nitrophenol (4-NP)

To evaluate the catalytic efficiency of 4-NP by the AgNPs prepared through the mentioned green synthetic method, we have prepared a 50 mM solution of 4-NP. As a hydrogen source, we prepared a 0.1 M solution of $NaBH_4$. When 15 mL of $NaBH_4$ solution is added to 15 mL of 4-NP solution, the color of the 4-NP solution turns to light yellow from light green indicating the formation of 4-nitrophenolate ions. As a blank experiment, we added only $NaBH_4$ to 4-NP and recorded UV-visible spectra at a regular time interval. To see the effect of catalyst AgNPs once we added both catalyst and $NaBH_4$ together and recorded its UV-visible spectra. In the first experiment of catalytic activity, we have added 1 mL of AgNPs extract, while in the other, we have added 2 mL of catalyst solution to observe the effect of catalyst amount variation in the reduction of 4-NP.

3. Results and Discussion

3.1. Biosynthesis and Characterization of AgNPs

3.1.1. Color Change and UV-Visible Spectroscopic Profile of Synthesized AgNPs

An apparent change in the color of the reaction mixture from light brown to dark brown after 30 min of incubation at room temperature in dark conditions was noticed in Figure 1. Indeed, no transformation in color was observed in $AgNO_3$ solution in the absence of plant extract under similar circumstances. The change in color was considered as an indication of AgNPs formation by the reduction of Ag^+ ions [35,56]. The formation of AgNPs was further confirmed by UV-Vis spectral study, which was measured at different reaction times (0.5, 1, 1.5, 2, 2.5 and 4 h, respectively) displayed in Figure 2a. The kinetics of the reaction revealed that the reaction was slow at the beginning, up to 30 min from the start of the reaction. After 30 min the nucleation of the reaction was initiated very quickly, and the formation of AgNPs occurred. This was reflected in the appearance of the characteristic band of AgNPs at ~430 nm after 30 min of reaction time (Figure 2a). The reaction was allowed to continue further, and no significant change of the peak was observed in the intensity of Ag peak, which exhibits towards the completion of the reaction at ~2.5 h. The broad absorption peak at $\lambda = 430$ nm represents the characteristics of surface plasmon resonance (SPR) of spherical and aggregate AgNPs formation [11]. The stability of the green synthesized AgNPs with respect to time was checked by UV-Vis spectroscopy after 1 day and 60 days. The characteristic $\lambda = 430$ nm peak was found in the synthesized AgNPs, indicating the stability of the synthesized AgNPs (Figure 2b). Thus, from this result, we can conclude that the synthesized AgNPs showed high aqueous stability since a minor reduction in absorbance was observed at 430 nm. A similar type of analysis with almost the same range of results was obtained previously in recent studies of green synthesis of AgNPs using extracts of different plants, such as pomegranate leaves, *Benincasa hispida*, *Prosopis juliflora*, *Allium cepa*, *Parkia speciosa* and *Salvia hispanica* [15,36,39,57–59].This suggests that the phytochemicals present in *Diospyros malabarica* fruit extracted successfully act as reducing and capping agents.

3.1.2. TEM

The size and morphology of green synthesized AgNPs were evaluated by TEM analysis. Figure 3a displays the SAED pattern of synthesized AgNPs, whereas Figure 3b demonstrates the spherical shape of the synthesized AgNPs and Figure 3c showed the particle size distribution of the AgNPs. The synthesized nanoparticles are polydisperse and range in size from 8 to 28 nm with an average size of 17.4 nm. The selected area electron diffraction (SAED) pattern displayed in Figure 3a of the AgNPs with bright spots indicated the polycrystalline nature of synthesized AgNPs, and each of their diffraction rings has been indexed to 111 and 220, the corresponding face-centered cubic (fcc)crystalline structure of metallic silver, which matches with the database of Joint Committee on Powder Diffraction Standards (JCPDS, No. 04-0783). The results of SAED were in congruence with the XRD pattern. Our analysis of SAED was almost similar to previously obtained results in some green synthesized AgNPs [11,60]. Our findings followed previous reports, where plant extract as a reducing agent was utilized in the synthesis of AgNPs, and almost similar results have been reported for AgNPs with the size of a nanoparticle ranging from 2 to 75 nm [61–63]. Due to this ultra-small size, shape and high stability, these synthesized AgNPs can be used in conjugating drugs and for targeting cancerous cells [56,64].

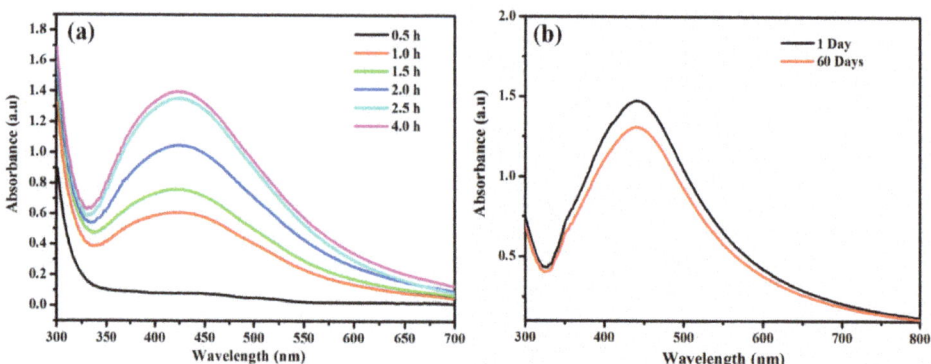

Figure 2. (a) UV-visible absorbance spectra kinetic reaction of the green synthesized AgNPs during the preparations at different time intervals. (b) UV-Vis spectra showing the stability of green synthesized AgNPs after 1 day and 60 days of preparation.

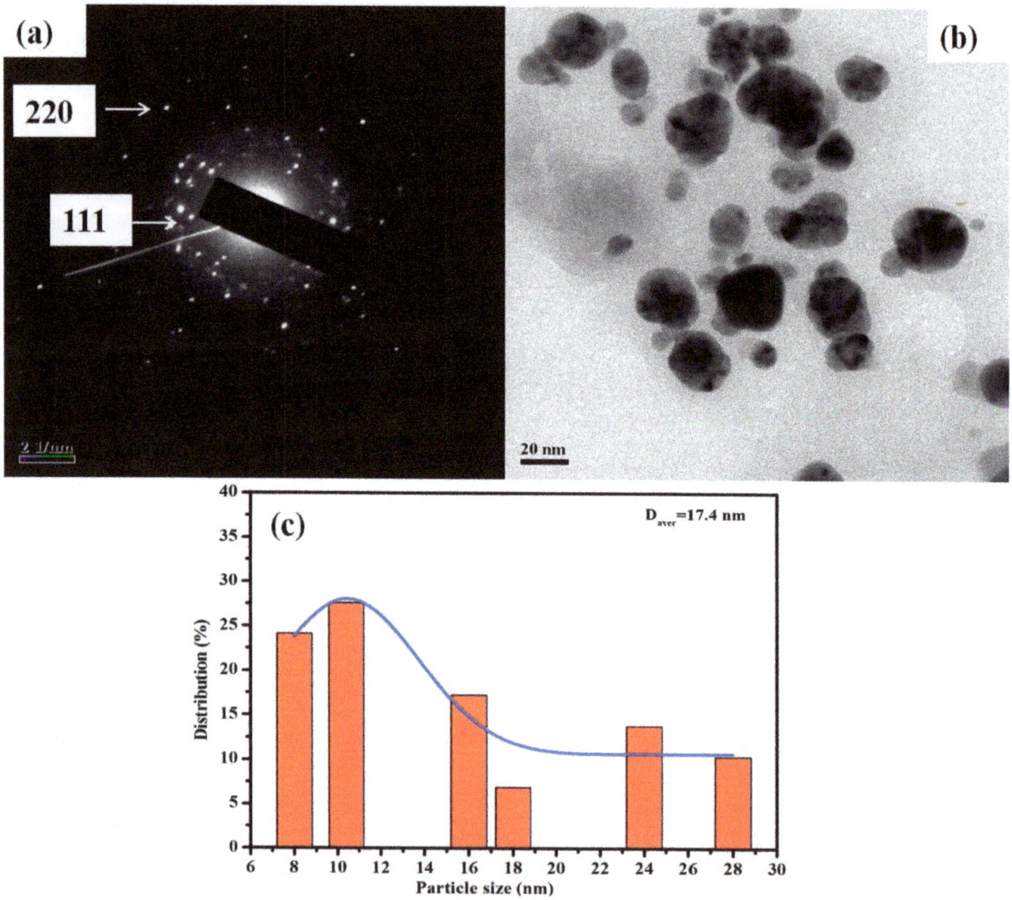

Figure 3. TEM micrograph of the synthesized AgNPs. (a) SAED pattern of synthesized AgNPs. (b) Analysis of the morphology of AgNPs. (c) Histogram showing the size distribution of AgNPs.

3.1.3. FESEM and EDX Analysis

Morphological characteristics of green synthesized AgNPs were determined by FE-SEM techniques. FESEM images of synthesized AgNPs were predominantly found to show spherical morphology with an average size of 48.72 nm (Figure 4a). The results evidently display that synthesized AgNPs material contains small grain-like particles, which were agglomerated to form crystals with an almost uniform spherical shape with a smooth surface (Figure 4a). A similar type of findings was previously reported [65–67]. Figure 4b displayed the EDAX spectrum of synthesized AgNPs, which describes the elemental analysis of the material. Silver peaks are seen in the spectrum, which represents the presence of silver ions as an ingredient element in the synthesized AgNPs. The Ag peak showed a weight percentage of 17.25 and an atomic percentage of 4.21. Other peaks, such as O, Na, Al, Cl, K, were observed. These elements were originated from the biomolecules present in the *Diospyros malabarica* fruit extract that was bound to the surface of the AgNPs. Strong Si peaks were observed due to the use of a glass coverslip where the samples were loaded, whereas Au peaks are due to gold sputtering during FESEM analysis. Our finding results were almost in agreement with previous findings [45,68,69].

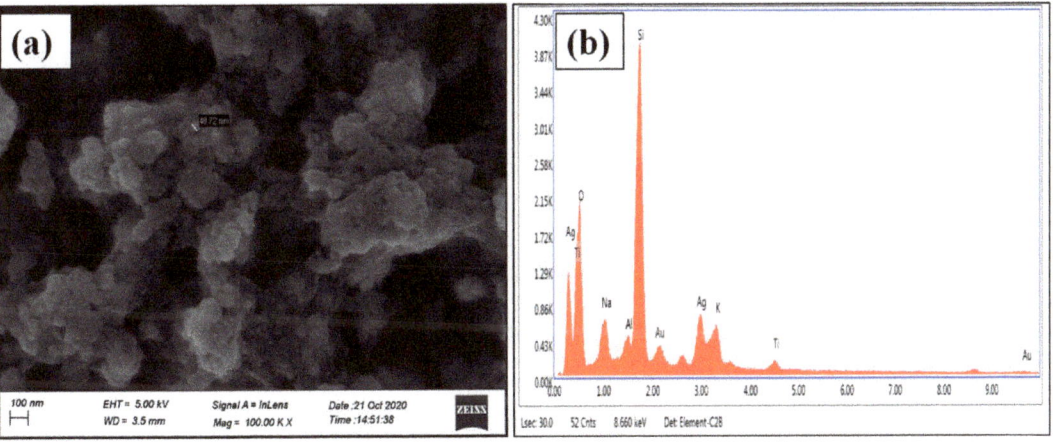

Figure 4. (**a**) FESEM recorded at the scale of 100 nm and (**b**) EDX image of synthesized AgNPs.

3.1.4. Particle Size and Zeta Potential (ζ) Analysis

The synthesized AgNPs were subjected to DLS and Zeta potential (ζ) measurement techniques for the analysis of size, PDI and surface charge of the nanoparticles. Particle size analysis showed two peaks, one of 22.26 nm and another of 1.032 nm, respectively, with PDI 0.954 (Figure 5a). This showed the polydispersity nature of our synthesized AgNPs. The stability and surface charge of the AgNPs was determined by zeta potential. It showed that the synthesized AgNPs were negatively charged with a zeta potential (mV) of -22.3 mV (Figure 5b). The results exhibit that the surface of the synthesized AgNPs was negatively charged, thereby having good colloidal nature, as well as well dispersed in the medium due to strong repulsion among the particles to evade the agglomeration [38]. The size of the green synthesized AgNPs was found nearly similar between the TEM and DLS analysis. The higher negativity value of the zeta potential specified stability and well-dispersed behavior of nanoparticles [70]. Thus, our results prove the efficacy of components present in the *Diospyros malabarica* fruit extract as reducing and capping agents for the synthesis of AgNPs.

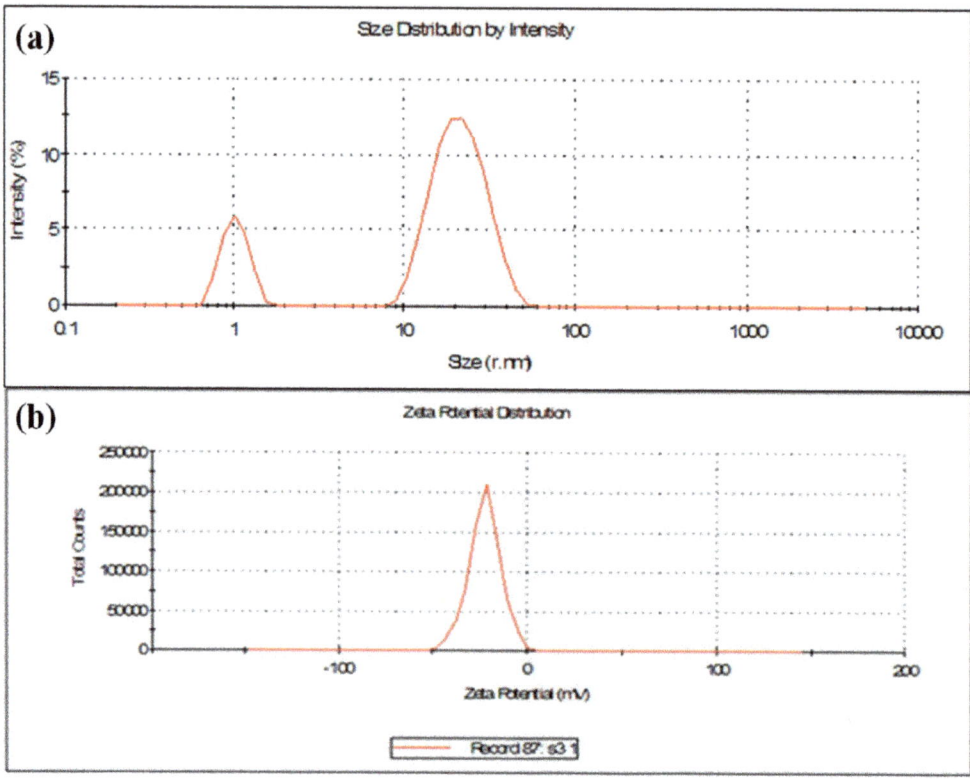

Figure 5. (a) Dynamic light scattering (DLS) and (b) zeta potential analysis of synthesized AgNPs.

3.1.5. XRD Analysis

The exact nature of the silver nanoparticles can be attained from XRD analysis. The XRD patterns of green synthesized AgNPs from fruit extract in Figure 6 showed Bragg's model diffraction peaks at 2θ on 32.1° and 64.4°, respectively. The peaks corresponding to the 2θ = 32.1° and 64.4° depicted (111) and (220) lattice planes for silver confirmed the face-centered cubic (FCC) crystalline nature of the AgNPs. This result corroborated with the XRD analysis reported earlier [61,71–73]. The diffraction patterns showed good agreement with JCPDS (no. 04-0783). Thus, XRD patterns clearly showed the crystalline AgNPs formed by the complete reduction of Ag^+ ions by the aqueous fruit extract of *Diospyros malabarica*. The other unassigned peak ensued the crystallization of silver nanoparticles along with the organic moieties or impurities that bound to the surface of nanoparticles [74–76]. The d spacing values were calculated from the theta values diffraction patterns using the following formula:

$$d = \lambda / 2 \sin \theta$$

where λ is the wavelength (0.154 nm) of X-rays, and θ is Bragg's angle of diffraction. The d spacing values were found to be d = 0.28 and 0.14 nm, respectively, which also corroborated with the (111) and (220) planes for silver nanoparticles.

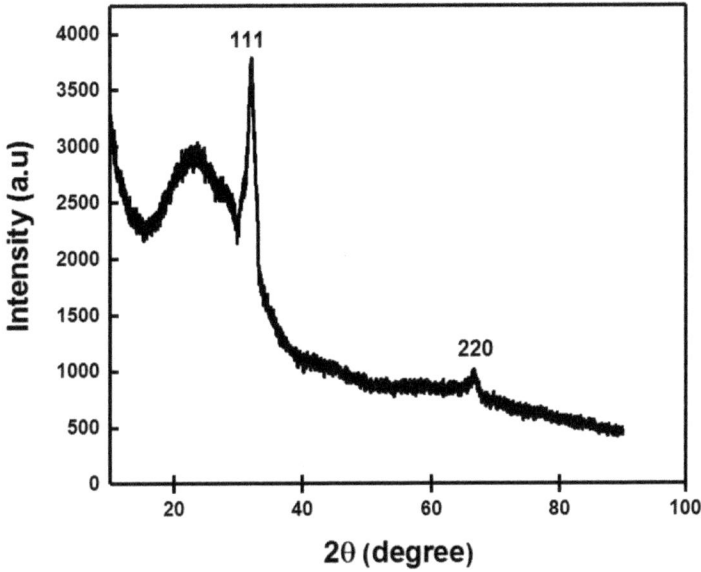

Figure 6. X-ray diffraction (XRD) pattern of green synthesized AgNPs.

3.1.6. FTIR Spectroscopy Analysis

FTIR spectroscopy analysis was conducted in order to determine the functional group of *Diospyros malabarica* fruit extract that was involved in the green synthesis of AgNPs as reducing and capping agents. Figure 7 displayed the FTIR spectral bands of the *Diospyros malabarica* fruit extract and synthesized AgNPs from the fruit extract. Sharp transmittance peaks were noticed at 3435, 2078, 1642, 1382 and 671 cm^{-1} in the synthesized AgNPs. As displayed in Figure 7, the FT-IR spectrum of *Diospyros malabarica* aqueous fruit extracts was closely similar to the FT-IR spectrum of the synthesized AgNPs, with a marginal shift in peaks. This similarity plainly indicates that some of the residual moieties of the phytochemicals present in the *Diospyros malabarica* fruit extract reside on the surface of the synthesized AgNPs. The FT-IR spectrum of *Diospyros malabarica* aqueous fruit extracts exhibits several absorption peaks at 3411, 2088, 1645, 1382 and 656 cm^{-1}, which are associated with several functional groups. Sharp transmittance peaks were also noticed at 3435, 2078, 1642, 1382 and 671 cm^{-1} in the synthesized AgNPs. The FT-IR spectrum peaks evidently indicate the role of *Diospyros malabarica* aqueous fruit extracts as reducing and stabilizing agents. The strong occurrence of intense peaks at 3411 and 3435 cm^{-1} was an indication of O–H stretching vibration type of hydroxyl and amine (N–H) functional groups. The absorbance peaks located between 3000 and 3600 cm^{-1} were assigned to the stretching vibrations of hydroxyl groups (O–H) and amine (N–H) [2]. O–H stretching vibration was characteristic of polyphenols and N–H stretching was attributed to the presence of amino acids, peptides and proteins [22,77]. The phenolic group of compounds present in the fruit extract has been shown as powerful capping and reducing agents for the formation of AgNPs by reduction of silver nitrate. More intense peaks were observed at 2088 and 2078 cm^{-1}, represented the presence of alkynes C≡C stretched vibration because of numerous secondary metabolites dissolved in the sample. The peaks at 1645 and 1642 cm^{-1} are attributed to the amide I band and –C=C– stretching vibration band. The 1382 cm^{-1} peak was attributed to the –C–N– stretching band as well as the amide I band of proteins in the fruit extract [45]. The amide band I was associated with the stretch mode of the carbonyl group (C=O) united to the amide linkage. The peaks at 656 and 671 cm^{-1} were assigned to CH out of plane bending vibrations [56]. This amide I band might also be due to the presence of proteins from the fruit extract [39,65]. The proteins might be capped or coated around the synthesized AgNPs for their stability and to prevent agglomeration [56]. Thus from the FTIR investigation, it was evident that bioactive compounds, such as polyphenols, along with proteins present in the *Diospyros malabarica* fruit extracts play an important role in the synthesis of AgNPs.

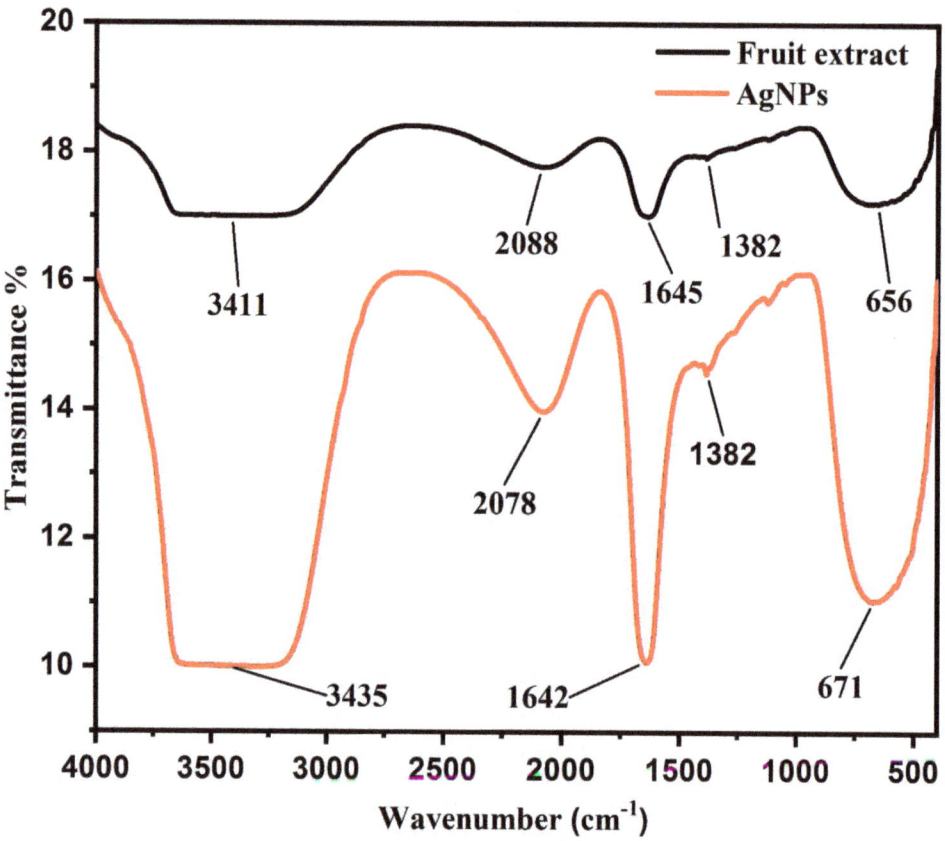

Figure 7. FTIR spectral analysis of *Diospyros malabarica* aqueous fruit extract and synthesized AgNPs.

3.1.7. Photoluminescence (PL) Studies

The photoluminescence (PL) of the synthesized AgNPs by *Diospyros malabarica* aqueous fruit extract was analyzed by fluorescence emission spectroscopy to analyze its optical property. The PL study showed the luminescence spectrum of the synthesized AgNPs at room temperature. The visible luminescence of AgNPs is due to the recombination of electron-hole pairs between d-band and sp-conduction above the Fermi level [78]. The synthesized AgNPs were dispersed in water, and the PL emission spectra were recorded at the different excitation wavelengths. The normalized fluorescence spectra of synthesized AgNPs were shown in Figure 8a. This illustrated that the AgNPs solution was irradiated at varieties of excitation wavelengths ranging from 320 to 430 nm, which showed different emission intensities centered at 470 nm. The fluorescence emission spectra were recorded at a fixed slit width of 5 nm. Thus, emission possesses an excitation wavelength-independent emission property. The literature reveals that the excitation independent properties are achieved by nanoparticles (NPs) due to doping or the presence of heteroatoms present on the surface of nanoparticles [79]. The normalized absorption and emission spectra of green synthesized AgNPs are shown in Figure 8b. It was observed that there was little overlap of absorption and emission spectra having large Stokes shift ($\Delta\lambda$ = 249.05 nm, or $\Delta\nu$ = 8884.15 cm^{-1}) in comparison to some of the commercial fluorescent dyes, such as fluorescein ($\Delta\lambda$ = 24 nm, or $\Delta\nu$ = 938 cm^{-1}) and Rhodamine 6G ($\Delta\lambda$ = 24 nm, or $\Delta\nu$ = 823 cm^{-1}) [80]. Such a large stokes shift helps to reduce self-quenching that occurs from molecular self-absorption. This instead makes the material useful in practical applications. The PL-quantum yield (QY) of AgNPs was measured following a standard procedure [81]. A comparison was made for integrated photoluminescence intensities (excited at 360 nm) and absorbance values (at 330 nm) using quinine sulfate (in 0.1 M H_2SO_4) as a standard (Φ = 0.54). The synthesized AgNPs and quinine sulfate were diluted to different concentrations so that it gives an absorbance below 0.1 at 330 nm. Then the PL-QY was calculated using the following equation.

$$\Phi_x = \Phi_{ST} \times (G_x \times G_{ST}) \times (\eta_x^2/\eta_{ST}^2)$$

Here G is the gradient of the plot, η is the refractive index of the solvent, Φ is the quantum yield while X refers to AgNPs, and ST refers to quinine sulfate with a refractive index of 1.33. Thus, a moderate quantum yield (0.06%) was found for the synthesized AgNPs. The plot of integrated fluorescence intensity versus absorbance was depicted in Figure 8c. The AgNPs in aqueous solution emits blue light, which is confirmed by CIE 1931 chromaticity parameters (x, y) calculated using CIE 1931 app [82], as shown in Figure 8d. We found CIE parameters for synthesized AgNPs solution as x = 0.21 and y = 0.54 when photo-excited at 430 nm that receives color temperature 8087.76 K. The triangle in the chromaticity plot represents the emission of blue light by AgNPs on excitation, which is in agreement with the normalized fluorescence spectra shown in Figure 8a. Thus, the synthesized AgNPs with optical properties can be utilized for bioimaging processes [83].

3.2. Antibacterial Activity of AgNPs

In the present investigation, the antibacterial effect of green synthesized AgNPs was subjected to evaluation on human pathogenic microorganisms *Escherichia coli* (Gram-negative) and *Staphylococcus aureus* (Gram-positive) by the agar well diffusion method (Figure 9). The antibacterial activities of *Diospyros malabarica* aqueous fruit extracts were also studied. Double distilled water (ddH_2O) was kept as a negative control and antibiotics (Streptomycin 10 µg, Tetracycline 30 µg and Chloramphenicol 30 µg) as a positive control. The zone of inhibition around the samples of individual bacterial cultures is shown in Figure 9a–h. Significant inhibition zone was observed in both the microbes on treatment with AgNPs. The zone of inhibition was measured to be 8.4 ± 0.3 and 12.1 ± 0.5 mm at 500 µg/mL and 1000 µg/mL concentrations of AgNPs, respectively, against *Staphylococcus aureus*. While in the case of *Escherichia coli*, it was measured to be 6.1 ± 0.7 and 13.1 ± 0.5 mm at a concentration of 500 and 1000 µg/mL AgNPs, respectively. Lesser antibacterial activity was observed in the case of *Diospyros malabarica* fruit extracts (*Escherichia coli*; 5 ± 0.5 mm) (*Staphylococcus aureus*; 7 ± 0.8 mm) in comparison to AgNPs in both the microorganisms. These results were almost similar to the previous report studied on the antibacterial activity of synthesized AgNPs using leaf extract of *Diospyrosmalabarica* [84]. On the other hand, the negative control did not exhibit any antibacterial activity. All the three standard antibiotics used as positive control were found to be moderate to highly sensitive against *E. coli* and *S. aureus*. The zone of inhibition against these two bacterial strains was recorded as Streptomycin 10 µg: 14 and 12 mm, Tetracycline 30 µg: 32 and 34 mm and Chloramphenicol 30 µg: 31 and 33 mm, respectively. It was clearly observed that the green synthesized AgNPs displayed concentration-dependent antibacterial activity. The zone of inhibition of synthesized AgNPs was almost comparable to streptomycin but smaller when compared to the other two antibiotics used. However, the as-synthesized AgNPs displayed a considerable antibacterial activity against both of the strains. This antibacterial activity of green synthesized AgNPs might be due to their penetration through the bacterial cell wall that caused the structural damage by interacting with sulfur and phosphorous-containing biomolecules. This has also generated free radicals, which in turn damage the bacterial membrane on contact with them [82]. The inhibitory zone on both of the microbes was accredited on treatment with aqueous fruit extracts of *Diospyros malabarica* due to the presence of phytochemicals, such as flavonoids, alkaloids and polyphenols. Whereas the antimicrobial effect of $AgNO_3$ was due to inhibition of proteins by binding with the thiol groups and also by binding with DNA, thereby arresting replication in bacteria as reported in earlier findings [84]. Previously, several studies reported the strong antimicrobial activity of silver nanoparticles synthesized from plant extracts. These AgNPs effectively killed a wide range of pathogenic microorganisms, e.g., *E. coli*, *S. aureus* and *P. aeruginosa* [85,86]. Our synthesized AgNPs possessed comparatively higher antimicrobial activity, as reported earlier by other workers [36,37]. Based on this experiment, synthesized AgNPs were found to have significant antibacterial efficacy against *Escherichia coli* and *Staphylococcus aureus*. The antimicrobial properties of these synthesized AgNPs may thus be utilized for medical, cosmetic and food industries.

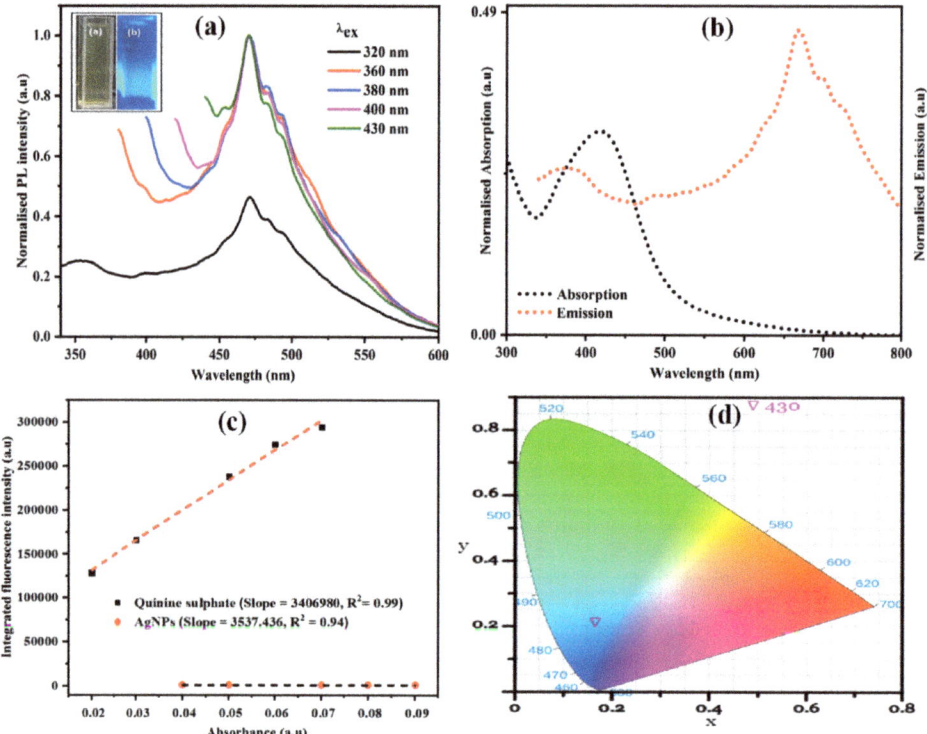

Figure 8. (a) Excitation-independent fluorescence emission spectra of green synthesized AgNPs (inset: AgNPs under (a) visible light, (b) UV light). (b) Absorption and emission spectra of green synthesized AgNPs. (c) Plot for calculation of quantum yield of AgNPs using quinine sulfate as standard. (d) Placement of the AgNPs fluorescence emission spectra on the CIE 1931 chromaticity chart.

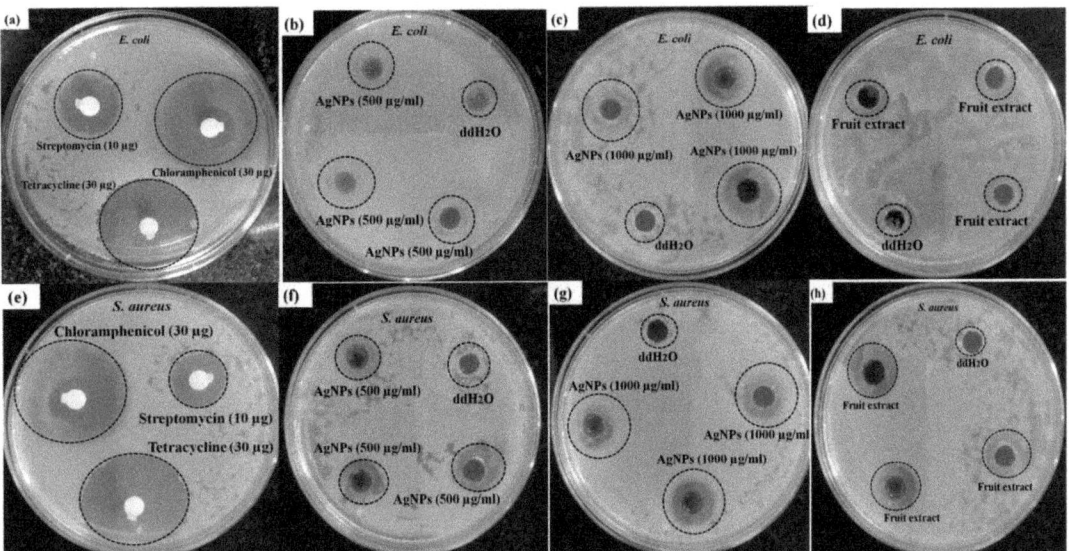

Figure 9. Antibacterial activities of (**a**,**e**) antibiotics (streptomycin(10 µg), Chloramphenicol (30 µg) and Tetracycline (30 µg)) as positive control, (**b**,**f**) synthesized AgNPs (500 µg/mL),(**c**,**g**) synthesized AgNPs (1000 µg/mL), (**d**,**h**) *Diospyros malabarica* aqueous fruit extracts (1000 µg/mL) and double distilled water (ddH$_2$O) as negative control, on (**a**) Escherichia coli and (**b**) Staphylococcus aureus (all the experiments were performed in triplicates).

3.3. Cytotoxic Effect of AgNPs on U87-MG Cells

To check the antiproliferative activity of the *Diospyros malabarica* fruit extract mediated green synthesized AgNPs, different concentrations (0, 10, 20, 40, 60, 80 and 100 µg/mL) of nanoparticles were added to U87-MG cancer cell lines and incubated for 48 h. The results were analyzed by MTT assay, which showed a decrease in viable cells with an increasing concentration of AgNPs (Figure 10). The IC$_{50}$ value of AgNPs was calculated to be 58.63 ± 5.74 µg/mL. Similar results were obtained from silver nanoparticles for U87MG cells reported earlier [87,88]. Green synthesized AgNPs using *Artemisia turcomanica* leaf extract also showed an IC$_{50}$ value close to 4.88 and 14.56 µg/mL for AGS and L-929 cells [89]. Biosynthesized AgNPs using *Cucumis prophetarum* aqueous leaf extract also showed antiproliferative activity against A549, MDA-MB-231, HepG2 and MCF-7 cell lines with IC$_{50}$ values of AgNPs 105.8, 81.1, 94.2 and 65.6 µg/mL, respectively [71]. The green synthesized AgNPs were found to be toxic in only cancerous cell lines and have negligible toxicity in normal cell lines [90,91]. The AgNPs also reported being capable of reducing various cell lines, such as HeLa, HepG2, PC3 and Vero cells [92,93]. The AgNPs with enhanced cytotoxicity tend to have high cellular uptake and retention via endocytosis and escaping efflux mechanism [88]. Further, at the IC$_{50}$ concentration of AgNPs, the morphology of the cells was observed under an inverted microscope (Figure 11). The untreated cells showed regular elongated cell structure while most of the cells appeared to be shrunken and formed round vesicular structures in the cells treated with AgNPs. The distorted cell morphology of cells treated with AgNPs may be attributed to the occurrence of apoptosis.

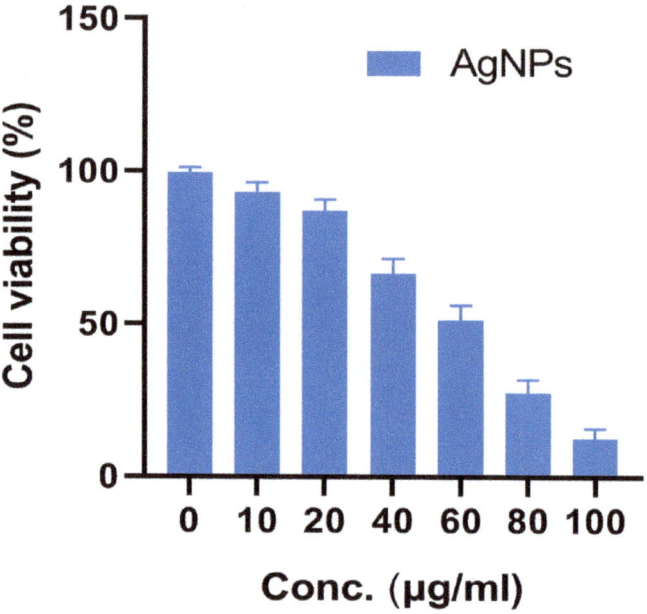

Figure 10. Effect of different concentrations of *Diospyros malabarica* extract mediated green synthesized AgNPs on the viability of U87-MG cell lines. Data represented as n = 3 ± S.D.

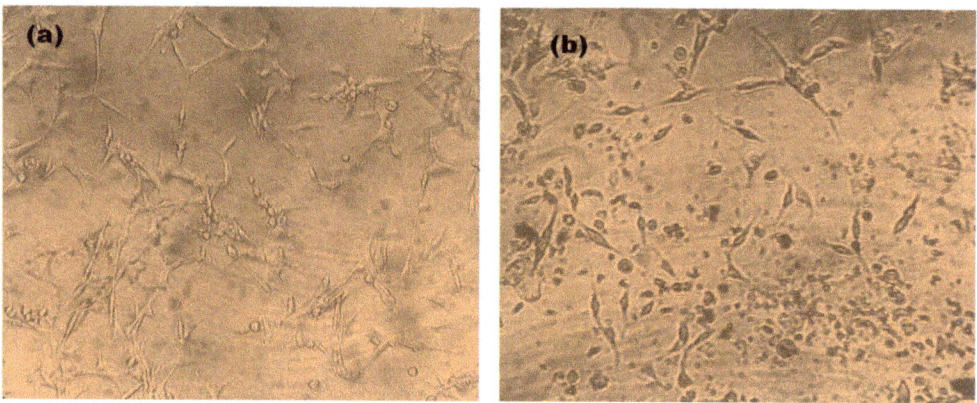

Figure 11. Cellular Morphology of U87-MG cells. (**a**) Untreated control, (**b**) *Diospyros malabarica* extract mediated green synthesized AgNPs treated at the IC$_{50}$ concentration.

3.4. Live/Dead Assay Analysis

To study the cell viability qualitative assessment of *Diospyros malabarica* fruit aqueous-extract-mediated green synthesized AgNPs, live/dead assays were performed on U87-MG cell lines (Figure 12). Thiazole orange (TO) and propidium iodide (PI) stains were selected as nucleic acid-binding dyes to observe live and dead cells under a confocal laser scanning microscope (CLSM). TO stains all live and dead cells as it is permeant to membrane, and PI stains only dead cells due to impermeability to live cells with intact cellular membranes. The images showed that the live cells had green color fluorescence (including dead cells), and dead cells had red color fluorescence. The untreated control cells revealed large numbers of live cells. On the other hand, the treated U87-MG cells with biosynthesized AgNPs depicted more apoptotic cells. The superimposed images divulged apprehension of the dead cells with a yellowish-orange and disfigured structure [3,94,95]. This result was in agreement with in vitro cytotoxicity assay (MTT analysis). The reduction of cell survival rate of U87-MG cells treated with AgNPs in MTT assay corroborated with the images obtained by LIVE/DEAD imaging that further aided in visualizing the live and dead cells treated by synthesized AgNPs.

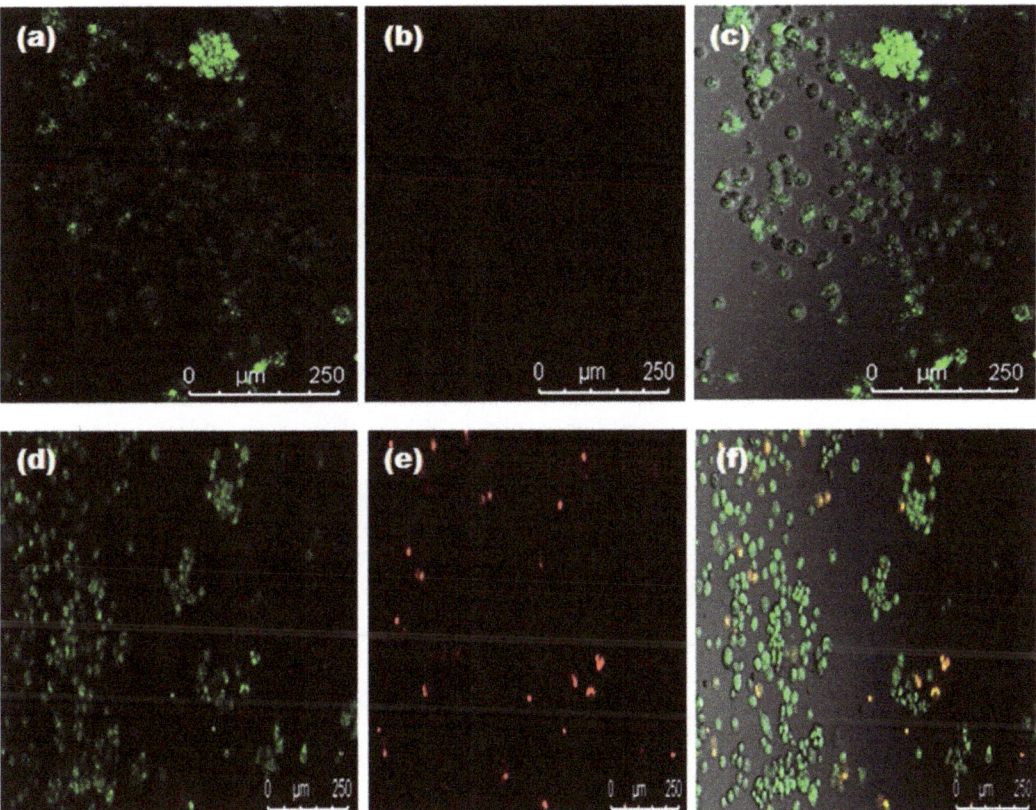

Figure 12. Confocal images of U87-MG cells at the IC_{50} concentration of *Diospyros malabarica* extract mediated green synthesized AgNPs incubated for 4 h. (**a**) TO, (**b**) PI, (**c**) superimposed image of untreated; (**d**) TO, (**e**) PI, (**f**) superimposed image treated with AgNPs.

3.5. Catalytic Reduction of 4-Nitrophenol (4-NP)

To see the catalytic efficiency of AgNPs, we used the reduction of 4-NP in the presence of $NaBH_4$ as a model reaction. The overall schematic representation for the reduction of 4-nitrophenol(4-NP) to 4-aminophenol (4-AP) was displayed in Figure 13. On the addition of $NaBH_4$ to 4-NP, it produced a 4-nitrophenolate ion. The 4-NP has a characteristic absorption at λ_{max} = 317 nm, while the 4-nitrophenolate ion absorbs at λ_{max} = 400 nm. On reduction of 4-NP to 4-AP, there would be a reduction of the peak at λ_{max} = 400 nm and the gradual appearance of a new peak at λ_{max} = 300 nm [26]. When we added 15 mL of 4-NP (50 mM) and 15 mL of $NaBH_4$ (0.1 M) and stirred continuously for one hour as a blank (control) experiment, we noticed the effect of only sodium borohydride ($NaBH_4$) in the reduction of 4-NP to 4-AP. There was a negligible change observed in the peak of 4-nitrophenolate at λ_{max} = 400 nm, as depicted in Figure 14a. However, on the addition of 1 mL of catalyst (AgNPs solution), we observed a continuous decrease in the λ_{max} of 4-nitrophenolate with the gradual appearance of a peak at 298–300 nm [24,26], as shown in Figure 14b. It was observed that within 15 min the 4-NP solution converted almost completely into 4-AP. In another similar experiment, we added an increased amount of catalyst. On the addition of 2 mL of AgNPs solution, 4-NP completely reduced within 5 min, as shown in Figure 14c. A plot C/C_0 versus time (in minutes) was plotted (Figure 14d) to compare the efficiency of NaBH$_4$ alone and various amounts of the catalyst with NaBH$_4$.

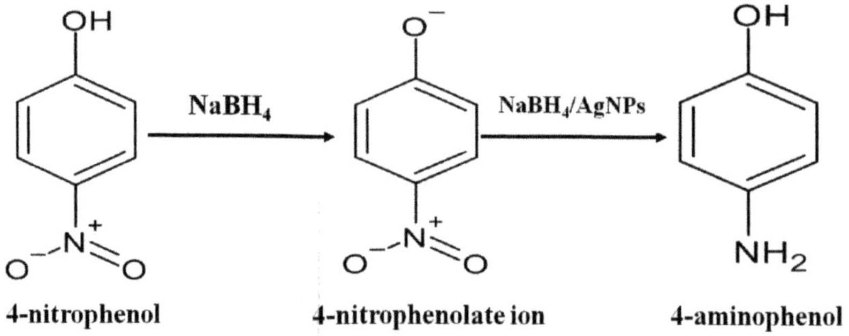

Figure 13. Schematic representation for reduction of 4-nitrophenol (4-NP) to 4-aminophenol (4-AP).

To study the kinetics of the reaction, a plot of $-\ln(C/C_0)$ was plotted as a function of time and was displayed in Figure 14e. The C/C_0 values were measured from the reduction of λ_{max} = 400 nm. The linear fit of the plot offered R-square values (coefficient of determination) 0.994 and 0.995, close to unity for a catalyst amount of 1 and 2 mL respectively. This supports the pseudo-first-order mechanism for the reduction of 4-NP. The apparent rate constants for the degradation of 4-NP by a catalyst amount of 1 and 2 mL were 0.20023 and 0.61127 min^{-1}, respectively, were calculated from the slopes. The appearance of the peak at 300 nm was an indication of the production of 4-AP. This investigation was further supported by the isosbestic points that emerged near 250, 270 and 325 nm that confirmed the 4-AP as the only product in the reaction [26].

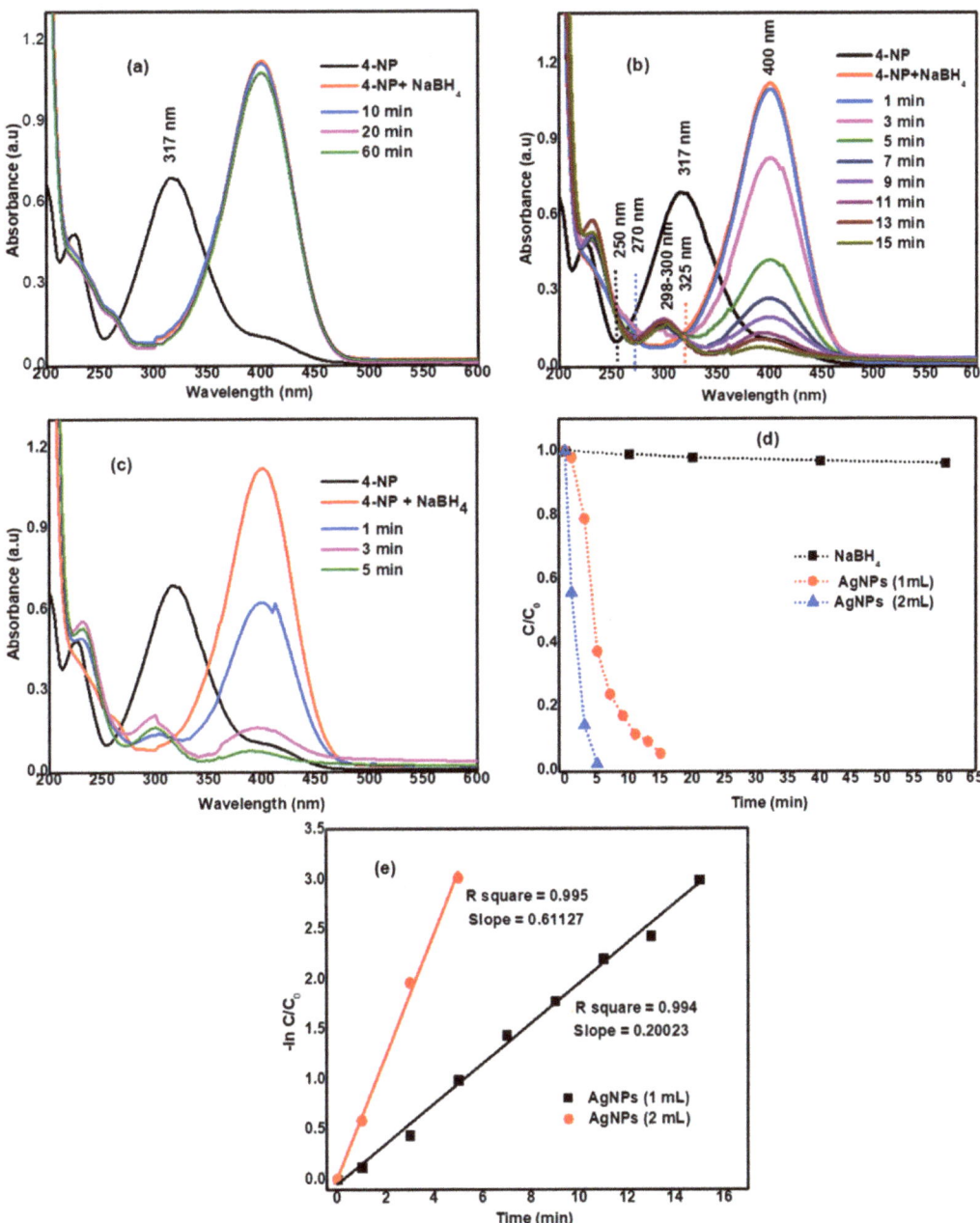

Figure 14. (a) Catalytic reduction of 4-NP by (a) NaBH$_4$, (b) 1 mL AgNPs, (c) 2 mL AgNPs, (d) C/C$_0$ and (e) −ln C/C$_0$ vs. time.

4. Conclusions

In the present investigation, we have successfully green synthesized AgNPs using an aqueous extract of *Diospyros malabarica* fruit. The method of preparation was simple, rapid, cost-effective and eco-friendly. The synthesized AgNPs were stable and smaller in size. The biomolecules present in the fruit, as well as proteins, contribute as a capping and reducing agent, which attributes to the synthesis of AgNPs. The biosynthesized AgNPs showed a significant antimicrobial effect against human pathogenic bacteria *Escherichia coli* and *Staphylococcus aureus*. The synthesized AgNPs exhibited significant dose-dependent anticancer activity on U87-MG (human primary glioblastoma) cells. Further, the synthesized AgNPs also act as a catalyst in the formation of 4-aminophenol by the reduction of 4-nitrophenol. 4-aminophenol has numerous applications in pharmaceutical industries, such as the production of antipyretic and analgesic drugs. Thus, the synthesized AgNPs showed their potential for implementations in cosmetics, therapeutics and food industries. However, in vivo experimental verification is required for its safe utilization.

Author Contributions: Conceptualization, D.B., K.K.B. and B.R.; methodology, K.K.B., B.R., B.K.C., N.K. and D.B.; formal analysis, K.K.B., B.R., T.S., S.K.G. and N.K.; investigation S.P., T.S. and K.K.B.; writing—original draft preparation, K.K.B., B.R., B.K.C. and S.P.; writing—review and editing, D.B., K.K.B., B.R., B.K.C., Z.A.K., S.K.G., H.A.E., S.P. and T.S. All authors have read and agreed to the published version of the manuscript.

Funding: No funding has been received from any funding agency to carry out the work. The APC for this publication was jointly supported by Universiti Sains Malaysia and Universiti Malaysia Kelantan.

Institutional Review Board Statement: Not applicable.

Data Availability Statement: Not applicable.

Acknowledgments: The authors acknowledge the aid for instrumentation facility in the Department of Applied Science, GUIST for FTIR; Sophisticated Analytical Instrument Facility, Gauhati University for XRD and FESEM.The authors also acknowledge Manos Pratim andChakrapaniKalita from the Department of Physics, Gauhati University, for providing the spectrofluorometer.

Conflicts of Interest: The authors declare no conflict of interest.

References

1. Mohanta, Y.K.; Nayak, D.; Biswas, K.; Singdevsachan, S.K.; Abd_Allah, E.F.; Hashem, A.; Alqarawi, A.A.; Yadav, D.; Mohanta, T.K. Silver nanoparticles synthesized using wild mushroom show potential antimicrobial activities against food borne pathogens. *Molecules* **2018**, *23*, 655. [CrossRef]
2. Hamouda, R.A.; Hussein, M.H.; Abo-elmagd, R.A.; Bawazir, S.S. Synthesis and biological characterization of silver nanoparticles derived from the cyanobacterium *Oscillatoria limnetica*. *Sci. Rep.* **2019**, *9*, 13071. [CrossRef] [PubMed]
3. Rabha, B.; Bharadwaj, K.K.; Baishya, D.; Sarkar, T.; Edinur, H.A.; Pati, S. Synthesis and characterization of diosgenin encapsulated poly-ε-caprolactone-pluronic nanoparticles and its effect on brain cancer cells. *Polymers* **2021**, *13*, 1322. [CrossRef]
4. Govindarajan, M.; Rajeswary, M.; Veerakumar, K.; Muthukumaran, U.; Hoti, S.L.; Benelli, G. Green synthesis and characterization of silver nanoparticles fabricated using *Anisomeles indica*: Mosquitocidal potential against malaria, dengue and Japanese encephalitis vectors. *Exp. Parasitol.* **2016**, *161*, 40–47. [CrossRef]
5. Saratale, R.G.; Benelli, G.; Kumar, G.; Kim, D.S.; Saratale, G.D. Bio-fabrication of silver nanoparticles using the leaf extract of an ancient herbal medicine, dandelion (*Taraxacum officinale*), evaluation of their antioxidant, anticancer potential, and antimicrobial activity against phytopathogens. *Environ. Sci. Pollut. Res.* **2018**, *25*, 10392–10406. [CrossRef] [PubMed]
6. Schabes-Retchkiman, P.S.; Canizal, G.; Herrera-Becerra, R.; Zorrilla, C.; Liu, H.B.; Ascencio, J.A. Biosynthesis and characterization of Ti/Ni bimetallic nanoparticles. *Opt. Mater.* **2006**, *29*, 95–99. [CrossRef]
7. Yokoyama, K.; Welchons, D.R. The conjugation of amyloid beta protein on the gold colloidal nanoparticles' surfaces. *Nanotechnology* **2007**, *18*, 105101. [CrossRef]
8. Mali, S.C.; Dhaka, A.; Githala, C.K.; Trivedi, R. Green synthesis of copper nanoparticles using *Celastrus paniculatus* Willd. leaf extract and their photocatalytic and antifungal properties. *Biotechnol. Rep.* **2020**, *27*, e00518. [CrossRef]
9. Selim, Y.A.; Azb, M.A.; Ragab, I.; Abd El-Azim, M. Green synthesis of zinc oxide nanoparticles using aqueous extract of *Deverra tortuosa* and their cytotoxic activities. *Sci. Rep.* **2020**, *10*, 3445. [CrossRef]
10. Huq, M.A. Green synthesis of silver nanoparticles using *Pseudoduganella eburnea* MAHUQ-39 and their antimicrobial mechanisms investigation against drug resistant human pathogens. *Int. J. Mol. Sci.* **2020**, *21*, 1510. [CrossRef]
11. Kumar, B.; Smita, K.; Cumbal, L.; Debut, A. Green synthesis of silver nanoparticles using Andean blackberry fruit extract. *Saudi J. Biol. Sci.* **2017**, *24*, 45–50. [CrossRef]
12. Lahiri, D.; Nag, M.; Sheikh, H.I.; Sarkar, T.; Edinur, H.; Siddhartha, P.; Ray, R. Microbiologically synthesized nanoparticles and their role in silencing the biofilm signaling cascade. *Front. Microbiol.* 2021. [CrossRef]

13. Nag, M.; Lahiri, D.; Sarkar, T.; Ghosh, S.; Dey, A.; Edinur, H.A.; Pati, S.; Ray, R.R. Microbial fabrication of nanomaterial and its role in disintegration of exopolymeric matrices of biofilm. *Front. Chem.* **2021**, *9*, 690590. [CrossRef]
14. Baharara, J.; Namvar, F.; Mousavi, M.; Ramezani, T.; Mohamad, R. Anti-angiogenesis effect of biogenic silver nanoparticles synthesized using *Saliva officinalis* on chick chorioalantoic membrane (CAM). *Molecules* **2014**, *19*, 13498–13508. [CrossRef] [PubMed]
15. Ravichandran, V.; Vasanthi, S.; Shalini, S.; Shah, S.A.A.; Tripathy, M.; Paliwal, N. Green synthesis, characterization, antibacterial, antioxidant and photocatalytic activity of *Parkia speciosa* leaves extract mediated silver nanoparticles. *Results Phys.* **2019**, *15*, 102565. [CrossRef]
16. Chinnasamy, G.; Chandrasekharan, S.; Koh, T.W.; Bhatnagar, S. Synthesis, characterization, antibacterial and wound healing efficacy of silver nanoparticles from *Azadirachta indica*. *Front. Microbiol.* **2021**, *12*, 611560. [CrossRef]
17. Jain, N.; Jain, P.; Rajput, D.; Patil, U.K. Green synthesized plant-based silver nanoparticles: Therapeutic prospective for anticancer and antiviral activity. *Micro Nano Syst. Lett.* **2021**, *9*, 5. [CrossRef]
18. Ghojavand, S.; Madani, M.; Karimi, J. Green synthesis, characterization and antifungal activity of silver nanoparticles using stems and flowers of felty germander. *J. Inorg. Organomet. Polym. Mater.* **2020**, *30*, 2987–2997. [CrossRef]
19. El-Rafie, H.M.; Abdel-Aziz Hamed, M. Antioxidant and anti-inflammatory activities of silver nanoparticles biosynthesized from aqueous leaves extracts of four *Terminalia* species. *Adv. Nat. Sci. Nanosci. Nanotechnol.* **2014**, *5*, 035008. [CrossRef]
20. Yuan, Y.-G.; Zhang, S.; Hwang, J.-Y.; Kong, I.-K. Silver nanoparticles potentiates cytotoxicity and apoptotic potential of camptothecin in human cervical cancer cells. *Oxidative Med. Cell. Longev.* **2018**, *2018*, 6121328. [CrossRef]
21. Ishida, T. Anticancer activities of silver ions in cancer and tumor cells and DNA damages by Ag+-DNA base-pairs reactions. *MOJ Tumor Res.* **2017**, *1*, 8–16.
22. David, L.; Moldovan, B.; Vulcu, A.; Olenic, L.; Perde-Schrepler, M.; Fischer-Fodor, E.; Florea, A.; Crisan, M.; Chiorean, I.; Clichici, S.; et al. Green synthesis, characterization and anti-inflammatory activity of silver nanoparticles using European black elderberry fruits extract. *Colloids Surf. B. Biointerfaces* **2014**, *122*, 767–777. [CrossRef]
23. Shurpik, D.N.; Sevastyanov, D.A.; Zelenikhin, P.V.; Padnya, P.L.; Evtugyn, V.G.; Osin, Y.N.; Stoikov, I.I. Nanoparticles based on the zwitterionic pillar[5]arene and Ag(+): Synthesis, self-assembly and cytotoxicity in the human lung cancer cell line A549. *Beilstein J. Nanotechnol.* **2020**, *11*, 421–431. [CrossRef] [PubMed]
24. Yudha, S.S.; Falahudin, A.; Wibowo, R.H.; Hendri, J.; Wicaksono, D.O. Reduction of 4-nitrophenol mediated by silver nanoparticles synthesized using aqueous leaf extract of *Peronema canescens*. *Bull. Chem. React. Eng. Catal.* **2021**, *16*. [CrossRef]
25. Shimoga, G.; Palem, R.R.; Lee, S.-H.; Kim, S.-Y. Catalytic degradability of p-nitrophenol using ecofriendly silver nanoparticles. *Metals* **2020**, *10*, 1661. [CrossRef]
26. Deka, P.; Deka, R.C.; Bharali, P. In situ generated copper nanoparticle catalyzed reduction of 4-nitrophenol. *New J. Chem.* **2014**, *38*, 1789–1793. [CrossRef]
27. Khawas, P.; Dash, K.K.; Das, A.J.; Deka, S.C. Modeling and optimization of the process parameters in vacuum drying of culinary banana (Musa ABB) slices by application of artificial neural network and genetic algorithm. *Dry. Technol.* **2016**, *34*, 491–503. [CrossRef]
28. Crisan, C.M.; Mocan, T.; Manolea, M.; Lasca, L.I.; Tăbăran, F.-A.; Mocan, L. Review on Silver nanoparticles as a novel class of antibacterial solutions. *Appl. Sci.* **2021**, *11*, 1120. [CrossRef]
29. Padnya, P.; Gorbachuk, V.; Stoikov, I. The role of calix[n]arenes and pillar[n]arenes in the design of silver nanoparticles: Self-assembly and application. *Int. J. Mol. Sci.* **2020**, *21*, 1425. [CrossRef] [PubMed]
30. Mehmood, A.; Murtaza, G.; Bhatti, T.M.; Raffi, M.; Kausar, R. Antibacterial efficacy of silver nanoparticles synthesized by a green method using bark extract of *Melia azedarach* L. *J. Pharm. Innov.* **2014**, *9*, 238–245. [CrossRef]
31. Teimuri-mofrad, R.; Hadi, R.; Tahmasebi, B.; Farhoudian, S.; Mehravar, M.; Nasiri, R. Green synthesis of gold nanoparticles using plant extract: Mini-review. *Nanochem. Res.* **2017**, *2*, 8–19. [CrossRef]
32. Johnson, P.; Krishnan, V.; Loganathan, C.; Govindhan, K.; Raji, V.; Sakayanathan, P.; Vijayan, S.; Sathishkumar, P.; Palvannan, T. Rapid biosynthesis of *Bauhinia variegata* flower extract-mediated silver nanoparticles: An effective antioxidant scavenger and α-amylase inhibitor. *Artif. Cells Nanomed. Biotechnol.* **2018**, *46*, 1488–1494. [CrossRef]
33. Kumar, B.; Smita, K.; Cumbal, L.; Angulo, Y. Fabrication of silver nanoplates using *Nephelium lappaceum* (Rambutan) peel: A sustainable approach. *J. Mol. Liq.* **2015**, *211*, 476–480. [CrossRef]
34. Chand, K.; Cao, D.; Eldin Fouad, D.; Hussain Shah, A.; Qadeer Dayo, A.; Zhu, K.; Nazim Lakhan, M.; Mehdi, G.; Dong, S. Green synthesis, characterization and photocatalytic application of silver nanoparticles synthesized by various plant extracts. *Arab. J. Chem.* **2020**, *13*, 8248–8261. [CrossRef]
35. Shaik, M.R.; Khan, M.; Kuniyil, M.; Al-Warthan, A.; Alkhathlan, H.Z.; Siddiqui, M.R.H.; Shaik, J.P.; Ahamed, A.; Mahmood, A.; Khan, M.; et al. Plant-extract-assisted green synthesis of silver nanoparticles using *Origanum vulgare* L. extract and their microbicidal activities. *Sustainability* **2018**, *10*, 913. [CrossRef]
36. Swilam, N.; Nematallah, K.A. Polyphenols profile of pomegranate leaves and their role in green synthesis of silver nanoparticles. *Sci. Rep.* **2020**, *10*, 14851. [CrossRef]
37. Behravan, M.; Hossein Panahi, A.; Naghizadeh, A.; Ziaee, M.; Mahdavi, R.; Mirzapour, A. Facile green synthesis of silver nanoparticles using *Berberis vulgaris* leaf and root aqueous extract and its antibacterial activity. *Int. J. Biol. Macromol.* **2019**, *124*, 148–154. [CrossRef] [PubMed]

38. Elemike, E.E.; Onwudiwe, D.C.; Nundkumar, N.; Singh, M.; Iyekowa, O. Green synthesis of Ag, Au and Ag-Au bimetallic nanoparticles using *Stigmaphyllon ovatum* leaf extract and their in vitro anticancer potential. *Mater. Lett.* **2019**, *243*, 148–152. [CrossRef]
39. Soliman, W.E.; Khan, S.; Rizvi, S.M.; Moin, A.; Elsewedy, H.S.; Abulila, A.S.; Shehata, T.M. Therapeutic applications of biostable silver nanoparticles synthesized using peel extract of *Benincasa hispida*: Antibacterial and anticancer activities. *Nanomaterials* **2020**, *10*, 1954. [CrossRef]
40. Tyavambiza, C.; Elbagory, A.M.; Madiehe, A.M.; Meyer, M.; Meyer, S. The antimicrobial and anti-inflammatory effects of silver nanoparticles synthesised from *Cotyledon orbiculata* aqueous extract. *Nanomaterials* **2021**, *11*, 1343. [CrossRef] [PubMed]
41. Yasmin, S.; Nouren, S.; Bhatti, H.N.; Iqbal, D.N.; Iftikhar, S.; Majeed, J.; Mustafa, R.; Nisar, N.; Nisar, J.; Nazir, A.; et al. Green synthesis, characterization and photocatalytic applications of silver nanoparticles using *Diospyros lotus*. *Green Process. Synth.* **2020**, *9*, 87–96. [CrossRef]
42. Mukunthan, K.S.; Elumalai, E.K.; Patel, T.N.; Murty, V.R. Catharanthus roseus: A natural source for the synthesis of silver nanoparticles. *Asian Pac. J. Trop. Biomed.* **2011**, *1*, 270–274. [CrossRef]
43. Sathishkumar, P.; Preethi, J.; Vijayan, R.; Mohd Yusoff, A.R.; Ameen, F.; Suresh, S.; Balagurunathan, R.; Palvannan, T. Anti-acne, anti-dandruff and anti-breast cancer efficacy of green synthesised silver nanoparticles using *Coriandrum sativum* leaf extract. *J. Photochem. Photobiol. B* **2016**, *163*, 69–76. [CrossRef] [PubMed]
44. Moteriya, P.; Chanda, S. Synthesis and characterization of silver nanoparticles using *Caesalpinia pulcherrima* flower extract and assessment of their in vitro antimicrobial, antioxidant, cytotoxic, and genotoxic activities. *Artif. Cells Nanomed. Biotechnol.* **2017**, *45*, 1556–1567. [CrossRef]
45. Anandalakshmi, K.; Venugobal, J.; Ramasamy, V. Characterization of silver nanoparticles by green synthesis method using Pedalium murex leaf extract and their antibacterial activity. *Appl. Nanosci.* **2016**, *6*, 399–408. [CrossRef]
46. de Jesús Ruíz-Baltazar, Á.; Reyes-López, S.Y.; Larrañaga, D.; Estévez, M.; Pérez, R. Green synthesis of silver nanoparticles using a *Melissa officinalis* leaf extract with antibacterial properties. *Results Phys.* **2017**, *7*, 2639–2643. [CrossRef]
47. Arya, G.; Kumari, R.M.; Gupta, N.; Kumar, A.; Chandra, R.; Nimesh, S. Green synthesis of silver nanoparticles using *Prosopis juliflora* bark extract: Reaction optimization, antimicrobial and catalytic activities. *Artif. Cells Nanomed. Biotechnol.* **2018**, *46*, 985–993. [CrossRef]
48. Dehghanizade, S.; Arasteh, J.; Mirzaie, A. Green synthesis of silver nanoparticles using *Anthemis atropatana* extract: Characterization and in vitro biological activities. *Artif. Cells Nanomed. Biotechnol.* **2018**, *46*, 160–168. [CrossRef] [PubMed]
49. Sinha, B.N.; Bansal, S. A review of phytochemical and biological studies of *Diospyros* species used in folklore medicine of Jharkhand. *J. Nat. Remed.* **2008**, *8*, 11–17.
50. Shubhra, R.D.; Polash, S.A.; Saha, T.; Hasan, A.; Hossain, S.; Islam, Z.; Sarker, S.R. Investigation of the phytoconstituents and antioxidant activity of *Diospyros malabarica* fruit extracts. *Adv. Biosci. Biotechnol.* **2019**, *10*, 431–454. [CrossRef]
51. Saeb, A.T.M.; Alshammari, A.S.; Al-Brahim, H.; Al-Rubeaan, K.A. Production of silver nanoparticles with strong and stable antimicrobial activity against highly pathogenic and multidrug resistant bacteria. *Sci. World J.* **2014**, *2014*, 704708. [CrossRef] [PubMed]
52. Osibe, D.A.; Chiejina, N.V.; Ogawa, K.; Aoyagi, H. Stable antibacterial silver nanoparticles produced with seed-derived callus extract of *Catharanthus roseus*. *Artif. Cells Nanomed. Biotechnol.* **2018**, *46*, 1266–1273. [CrossRef]
53. Pati, S.; Chatterji, A.; Dash, B.P.; Nelson, B.R.; Sarkar, T.; Shahimi, S.; Edinur, H.A.; Abd Manan, T.S.B.; Jena, P.; Mohanta, Y.K.; et al. Structural characterization and antioxidant potential of chitosan by γ-irradiation from the carapace of horseshoe crab. *Polymers* **2020**, 2361. [CrossRef]
54. Pati, S.; Sarkar, T.; Sheikh, H.I.; Bharadwaj, K.K.; Mohapatra, P.K.; Chatterji, A.; Dash, B.P.; Edinur, H.A.; Nelson, B.R. γ-irradiated chitosan from *Carcinoscorpius rotundicauda* (Latreille, 1802) improves the shelf life of refrigerated aquatic products. *Front. Mar. Sci.* **2021**, *8*, 498. [CrossRef]
55. Balouiri, M.; Sadiki, M.; Ibnsouda, S.K. Methods for in vitro evaluating antimicrobial activity: A review. *J. Pharm. Anal.* **2016**, *6*, 71–79. [CrossRef]
56. Bethu, M.S.; Netala, V.R.; Domdi, L.; Tartte, V.; Janapala, V.R. Potential anticancer activity of biogenic silver nanoparticles using leaf extract of *Rhynchosia suaveolens*: An insight into the mechanism. *Artif. Cells Nanomed. Biotechnol.* **2018**, *46*, 104–114. [CrossRef] [PubMed]
57. Jini, D.; Sharmila, S. Green synthesis of silver nanoparticles from *Allium cepa* and its in vitro antidiabetic activity. *Mater. Today Proc.* **2020**, *22*, 432–438. [CrossRef]
58. Hernández-Morales, L.; Espinoza-Gómez, H.; Flores-López, L.Z.; Sotelo-Barrera, E.L.; Núñez-Rivera, A.; Cadena-Nava, R.D.; Alonso-Núñez, G.; Espinoza, K.A. Study of the green synthesis of silver nanoparticles using a natural extract of dark or white *Salvia hispanica* L. seeds and their antibacterial application. *Appl. Surf. Sci.* **2019**, *489*, 952–961. [CrossRef]
59. Arya, G.; Kumari, R.M.; Sharma, N.; Gupta, N.; Kumar, A.; Chatterjee, S.; Nimesh, S. Catalytic, antibacterial and antibiofilm efficacy of biosynthesised silver nanoparticles using *Prosopis juliflora* leaf extract along with their wound healing potential. *J. Photochem. Photobiol. B* **2019**, *190*, 50–58. [CrossRef] [PubMed]
60. Sangaonkar, G.M.; Pawar, K.D. Garcinia indica mediated biogenic synthesis of silver nanoparticles with antibacterial and antioxidant activities. *Colloids Surf. B Biointerfaces* **2018**, *164*, 210–217. [CrossRef]

61. Garibo, D.; Borbón-Nuñez, H.A.; de León, J.N.D.; García Mendoza, E.; Estrada, I.; Toledano-Magaña, Y.; Tiznado, H.; Ovalle-Marroquin, M.; Soto-Ramos, A.G.; Blanco, A.; et al. Green synthesis of silver nanoparticles using *Lysiloma acapulcensis* exhibit high-antimicrobial activity. *Sci. Rep.* **2020**, *10*, 12805. [CrossRef] [PubMed]
62. Salari, S.; Esmaeilzadeh Bahabadi, S.; Samzadeh-Kermani, A.; Yosefzaei, F. In-vitro evaluation of antioxidant and antibacterial potential of greensynthesized silver nanoparticles using *Prosopis farcta* fruit extract. *Iran. J. Pharm. Res. IJPR* **2019**, *18*, 430–455.
63. Jahan, I.; Erci, F.; Isildak, I. Microwave-assisted green synthesis of non-cytotoxic silver nanoparticles using the aqueous extract of *Rosa santana* (rose) petals and their antimicrobial activity. *Anal. Lett.* **2019**, *52*, 1860–1873. [CrossRef]
64. Karwa, A.; Gaikwad, S.; Rai, M.K. Mycosynthesis of silver nanoparticles using Lingzhi or Reishi medicinal mushroom, *Ganoderma lucidum* (W. Curt.:Fr.) P. Karst. and their role as antimicrobials and antibiotic activity enhancers. *Int. J. Med. Mushrooms* **2011**, *13*, 483–491. [CrossRef] [PubMed]
65. Ashokkumar, S.; Ravi, S.; Kathiravan, V.; Velmurugan, S. Synthesis, characterization and catalytic activity of silver nanoparticles using *Tribulus terrestris* leaf extract. *Spectrochim. Acta Part A Mol. Biomol. Spectrosc.* **2014**, *121*, 88–93. [CrossRef]
66. Venugobal, J.; Anandalakshmi, K. Green synthesis of silver nanoparticles using *Commiphora caudata* leaves extract and the study of bactericidal efficiency. *J. Clust. Sci.* **2016**, *27*, 1683–1699. [CrossRef]
67. Vinay, S.P.; Udayabhanu; Nagarju, G.; Chandrappa, C.P.; Chandrasekhar, N. Enhanced photocatalysis, photoluminescence, and anti-bacterial activities of nanosize Ag: Green synthesized via *Rauvolfia tetraphylla* (devil pepper). *SN Appl. Sci.* **2019**, *1*, 477. [CrossRef]
68. Ajitha, B.; Ashok Kumar Reddy, Y.; Sreedhara Reddy, P. Green synthesis and characterization of silver nanoparticles using *Lantana camara* leaf extract. *Mater. Sci. Eng. C* **2015**, *49*, 373–381. [CrossRef] [PubMed]
69. Gomathi, A.C.; Xavier Rajarathinam, S.R.; Mohammed Sadiq, A.; Rajeshkumar, S. Anticancer activity of silver nanoparticles synthesized using aqueous fruit shell extract of *Tamarindus indica* on MCF-7 human breast cancer cell line. *J. Drug Deliv. Sci. Technol.* **2020**, *55*, 101376. [CrossRef]
70. Govindan, L.; Anbazhagan, S.; Altemimi, A.B.; Lakshminarayanan, K.; Kuppan, S.; Pratap-Singh, A.; Kandasamy, M. Efficacy of antimicrobial and larvicidal activities of green synthesized silver nanoparticles using leaf extract of *Plumbago auriculata* Lam. *Plants* **2020**, *9*, 577. [CrossRef]
71. Hemlata; Meena, P.R.; Singh, A.P.; Tejavath, K.K. Biosynthesis of silver nanoparticles using *Cucumis prophetarum* aqueous leaf extract and their antibacterial and antiproliferative activity against cancer cell lines. *ACS Omega* **2020**, *5*, 5520–5528. [CrossRef]
72. Venkatadri, B.; Shanparvish, E.; Rameshkumar, M.R.; Arasu, M.V.; Al-Dhabi, N.A.; Ponnusamy, V.K.; Agastian, P. Green synthesis of silver nanoparticles using aqueous rhizome extract of *Zingiber officinale* and *Curcuma longa*: In-vitro anti-cancer potential on human colon carcinoma HT-29 cells. *Saudi J. Biol. Sci.* **2020**, *27*, 2980–2986. [CrossRef]
73. Zhang, X.-F.; Park, J.-H.; Choi, Y.-J.; Kang, M.-H.; Gurunathan, S.; Kim, J.-H. Silver nanoparticles cause complications in pregnant mice. *Int. J. Nanomed.* **2015**, *10*, 7057–7071. [CrossRef]
74. Awwad, A.M.; Salem, N.M.; Abdeen, A.O. Green synthesis of silver nanoparticles using carob leaf extract and its antibacterial activity. *Int. J. Ind. Chem.* **2013**, *4*, 29. [CrossRef]
75. Shanmuganathan, R.; MubarakAli, D.; Prabakar, D.; Muthukumar, H.; Thajuddin, N.; Kumar, S.S.; Pugazhendhi, A. An enhancement of antimicrobial efficacy of biogenic and ceftriaxone-conjugated silver nanoparticles: Green approach. *Environ. Sci. Pollut. Res. Int.* **2018**, *25*, 10362–10370. [CrossRef] [PubMed]
76. Pirtarighat, S.; Ghannadnia, M.; Baghshahi, S. Green synthesis of silver nanoparticles using the plant extract of *Salvia spinosa* grown in vitro and their antibacterial activity assessment. *J. Nanostruct. Chem.* **2019**, *9*, 1–9. [CrossRef]
77. Cheng, K.; Hung, Y.; Chen, C.; Liu, C.; Young, J. Green synthesis of chondroitin sulfate-capped silver nanoparticles: Characterization and surface modification. *Carbohydr. Polym.* **2014**, *110*, 195–202. [CrossRef]
78. Verma, A.; Mehata, M.S. Controllable synthesis of silver nanoparticles using Neem leaves and their antimicrobial activity. *J. Radiat. Res. Appl. Sci.* **2016**, *9*, 109–115. [CrossRef]
79. Bhati, A.; Anand, S.R.; Saini, D.; Khare, P.; Dubey, P.; Sonkar, S.K. Self-doped nontoxic red-emitting Mg–N-embedded carbon dots for imaging, Cu(ii) sensing and fluorescent ink. *New J. Chem.* **2018**, *42*, 19548–19556. [CrossRef]
80. Gao, Z.; Hao, Y.; Zheng, M.; Chen, Y. A fluorescent dye with large Stokes shift and high stability: Synthesis and application to live cell imaging. *RSC Adv.* **2017**, *7*, 7604–7609. [CrossRef]
81. Patir, K.; Gogoi, S.K. Facile synthesis of photoluminescent graphitic carbon nitride quantum dots for Hg^{2+} detection and room temperature phosphorescence. *ACS Sustain. Chem. Eng.* **2018**, *6*, 1732–1743. [CrossRef]
82. Hasabeldaim, E.H. CIE chromaticity diagram 1931 2021.
83. Francis, S.; Joseph, S.; Koshy, E.P.; Mathew, B. Microwave assisted green synthesis of silver nanoparticles using leaf extract of *Elephantopus scaber* and its environmental and biological applications. *Artif. Cells Nanomed. Biotechnol.* **2018**, *46*, 795–804. [CrossRef]
84. Taranath, T.; Hedaginal, B.; Rajani, P.; Sindhu, M. Phytosynthesis of silver nanoparticles using the leaf extract of *Diospyros malabarica* (desr.) Kostel and its antibacterial activity against human pathogenic gram negative *Escherichia coli* and *Pseudomonas aeruginosa*. *Int. J. Pharm. Sci. Rev. Res.* **2015**, *30*, 109–114.
85. Mohamed, D.S.; Abd El-Baky, R.M.; Sandle, T.; Mandour, S.A.; Ahmed, E.F. Antimicrobial activity of silver-treated bacteria against other multi-drug resistant pathogens in their environment. *Antibiotics* **2020**, *9*, 181. [CrossRef]

86. Javan bakht Dalir, S.; Djahaniani, H.; Nabati, F.; Hekmati, M. Characterization and the evaluation of antimicrobial activities of silver nanoparticles biosynthesized from *Carya illinoinensis* leaf extract. *Heliyon* **2020**, *6*, e03624. [CrossRef]
87. Loo, Y.Y.; Rukayadi, Y.; Nor-Khaizura, M.-A.-R.; Kuan, C.H.; Chieng, B.W.; Nishibuchi, M.; Radu, S. In vitro antimicrobial activity of green synthesized silver nanoparticles against selected gram-negative foodborne pathogens. *Front. Microbiol.* **2018**, *9*, 1555. [CrossRef]
88. Satpathy, S.; Patra, A.; Ahirwar, B.; Delwar Hussain, M. Antioxidant and anticancer activities of green synthesized silver nanoparticles using aqueous extract of tubers of *Pueraria tuberosa*. *Artif. Cells Nanomed. Biotechnol.* **2018**, *46*, S71–S85. [CrossRef] [PubMed]
89. Mousavi, B.; Tafvizi, F.; Zaker Bostanabad, S. Green synthesis of silver nanoparticles using *Artemisia turcomanica* leaf extract and the study of anti-cancer effect and apoptosis induction on gastric cancer cell line (AGS). *Artif. Cells Nanomed. Biotechnol.* **2018**, *46*, 499–510. [CrossRef]
90. Liu, X.; Shan, K.; Shao, X.; Shi, X.; He, Y.; Liu, Z.; Jacob, J.A.; Deng, L. Nanotoxic effects of silver nanoparticles on normal HEK-293 cells in comparison to cancerous HeLa cell line. *Int. J. Nanomed.* **2021**, *16*, 753–761. [CrossRef] [PubMed]
91. Kong, Y.; Paray, B.A.; Al-Sadoon, M.K.; Fahad Albeshr, M. Novel green synthesis, chemical characterization, toxicity, colorectal carcinoma, antioxidant, anti-diabetic, and anticholinergic properties of silver nanoparticles: A chemopharmacological study. *Arab. J. Chem.* **2021**, *14*, 103193. [CrossRef]
92. Sarkar, S.; Kotteeswaran, V. Green synthesis of silver nanoparticles from aqueous leaf extract of Pomegranate (*Punica granatum*) and their anticancer activity on human cervical cancer cells. *Adv. Nat. Sci. Nanosci. Nanotechnol.* **2018**, *9*, 025014. [CrossRef]
93. Prasannaraj, G.; Venkatachalam, P. Green engineering of biomolecule-coated metallic silver nanoparticles and their potential cytotoxic activity against cancer cell lines. *Adv. Nat. Sci. Nanosci. Nanotechnol.* **2017**, *8*, 025001. [CrossRef]
94. Hajrezaie, M.; Paydar, M.; Looi, C.Y.; Moghadamtousi, S.Z.; Hassandarvish, P.; Salga, M.S.; Karimian, H.; Shams, K.; Zahedifard, M.; Majid, N.A.; et al. Apoptotic effect of novel Schiff based $CdCl_2$ ($C_{14}H_{21}N_3O_2$) complex is mediated via activation of the mitochondrial pathway in colon cancer cells. *Sci. Rep.* **2015**, *5*, 9097. [CrossRef] [PubMed]
95. Rahbar Saadat, Y.; Saeidi, N.; Zununi Vahed, S.; Barzegari, A.; Barar, J. An update to DNA ladder assay for apoptosis detection. *Bioimpacts* **2015**, *5*, 25–28. [CrossRef]

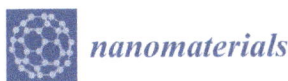

Article

Evaluation of Silica-Coated Insect Proof Nets for the Control of *Aphis fabae*, *Sitophilus oryzae*, and *Tribolium confusum*

Paraskevi Agrafioti [1,*], Sofia Faliagka [2], Evagelia Lampiri [1], Merle Orth [3], Mark Pätzel [3], Nikolaos Katsoulas [2] and Christos G. Athanassiou [1]

1. Laboratory of Entomology and Agricultural Zoology, Department of Agriculture, Crop Production and Rural Environment, University of Thessaly, Phytokou str., 38446 Volos, Magnesia, Greece; elampiri@agr.uth.gr (E.L.); athanassiou@agr.uth.gr (C.G.A.)
2. Laboratory of Agricultural Constructions and Environmental Control, Department of Agriculture Crop Production and Rural Environment, University of Thessaly, Phytokou Street, 38446 Volos Magnesia, Greece; sofia.faliagka@gmail.com (S.F.); nkatsoul@uth.gr (N.K.)
3. Institut für Textiltechnik der RWTH Aachen University, Otto-Blumenthal-St. 1, 52074 Aachen, Germany; merle.orth1@gmail.com (M.O.); mark.paetzel@ita.rwth-aachen.de (M.P.)
* Correspondence: agrafiot@agr.uth.gr

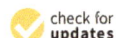

Received: 13 July 2020; Accepted: 18 August 2020; Published: 24 August 2020

Abstract: Insect proof nets are widely used in agriculture as mechanical and physical barriers to regulate pest populations in a greenhouse. However, their integration in the greenhouse ventilation openings is highly associated with the decrease of air flow and the adequate ventilation. Thus, there is need for alternative pest management tools that do not impair adequate ventilation. In the present study, we tested four net formulations of relatively large mesh size coated with SiO_2 nanoparticles, namely, ED3, ED3-P, ED5, and ED5-P to evaluate their insecticidal properties against adults of *Aphis fabae* and *Sitophilus oryzae* and larvae of *Tribolium confusum*. ED3 and ED5 nets were coated with SiO_2 nanoparticles of different diameter, while in the case of ED3-P and ED5-P, paraffin was added to increase the mass of the deposited particles on the net's surface. In the first series of bioassays, the knockdown and mortality rates of these species were evaluated after exposure to the aforementioned net formulations for 5, 10, 15, 20, 25, 30, 60, 90, and 180 min. In the second series of bioassays, knockdown and mortality of these species were recorded after 1, 7, and 10 days of post-exposure to the nets for different time intervals (15, 30, and 60 min). Based on our results, all nets significantly affected *A. fabae*, since all insects were dead at the 1-day post-exposure period to the silica-treated nets. Conversely, at the same interval, no effect on either *S. oryzae* adults or *T. confusum* larvae was observed. However, in the case of *S. oryzae*, the efficacy of all nets reached 100% 7 days after the exposure, even for adults that had been initially exposed for 15 min to the treated nets. Among the species tested, *T. confusum* larvae exhibited the lowest mortality rate, which did not exceed 34% at the 10 days of post-exposure interval. Our work underlines the efficacy of treated nets in pest management programs, under different application scenarios, at the pre- and post-harvest stages of agricultural commodities.

Keywords: net formulations; stored product insects; knockdown; mortality; long-term effect

1. Introduction

Despite the association of many insecticidal compounds with mammalian toxicity and increased environmental footprint, conventional pesticides are widely used as a means of pest management. Over the years, many insects species have developed resistance mechanisms to the vast majority of active ingredients that are used as synthetic insecticides [1–3]. According to the European Commission, a sustainable and environmentally friendly insecticidal strategy should be followed in the case of adequate crop protection, to minimize the negative effects of the intensive chemical pesticide applications on both natural enemies (predators, parasitoids) and human health [4,5]. Thus, the notion of integrated pest management (IPM) has now become entrenched in agriculture.

Nets are widely used in agriculture as mechanical or physical barriers in order to protect crops from either biotic or abiotic stresses. In the Mediterranean region, protection against insects is considered significantly important even compared to the management of excessive heat during the summer [6]. Insect proof nets have been integrated in greenhouse ventilation openings as an alternative to pesticides for many years and their use is related to the management of the population density of external agents. At the same time, exclusion nets are used to cover entire greenhouse structures or screenhouses [7]. Nets have a dual effect as they block the penetration of pests, while prevent the escape of insects used for crop pollination [8]. The design of nettings is determined by the size and geometry of the hole, the size of the insect thorax, as well as the method of knitting [9].

According to Kittas et al. [6], the environment of a greenhouse is qualified by significant heterogeneity in which various factors contribute, such as the crop itself, the cover materials and the insect screens. Microclimate conditions of a greenhouse are strongly affected by nets' physical and optical properties [10]. Very fine mesh size nets severely affect the ventilation and air capacity of the enclosed area by decreasing permeability [11,12]. Indeed, the ventilation rate can be decreased by 40–50% when anti-aphid or anti-thrip nettings are applied [11,13]. These results are in accordance with those of Katsoulas et al. [14], who indicated a 33% decrease of ventilation flow due to the installation of an anti-aphid insect screen with 50% porosity on the vents of a polyethylene-covered greenhouse. In addition, Baeza et al. [15] showed that the use of an anti-insect screen with porosity of 25%, which is commonly used to exclude white flies *Bemisia tabaci* (Gennadius) (Hemiptera: Aleyrodoidae) and the western flower thrips *Frankliniella occidentalis* (Pergande) (Thysanoptera: Thripidae), could lead to a ventilation reduction of approximately 88%. As a result, higher temperature regimes are recorded in the interior of the protected greenhouse plants leading to non-uniform production, increased yield losses, as well as quality deterioration [6,14]. Small mesh size nets (i.e., low porosity nets) may contribute to undesired results, since they exclude not only harmful pests but also beneficial insects [16]. Moreover, Bell and Baker [11], showed that the migration of insects in a greenhouse is not always correlated to the mesh size, since insects with very small thoracic width, such as whiteflies, can intrude the finest pore size net.

The establishment of insect proof nets for the stored product pest management is directly linked to environmental protection, as their use does not lead to residues or to contamination in storage facilities and stored commodities [17]. Many studies are focused on the design of long-lasting insecticide-treated nets (LLINs) by incorporating insecticides into the net coating in order to minimize the chemical sprays directly on the crop [18,19]. Dáder et al. [18] showed that LLINs caused a significant reduction in *Myzus persicae* (Sulzer) (Hemipetra: Aphidedae) and *Aphis gossypii* (Glover) (Hemipetra: Aphididae) immigration without affecting the parasitoid *Aphidius colemani* Viereck (Hymenoptrea: Aphididae). However, during field trials, LLINs effectiveness was degraded after sun exposure whereas, the efficacy of either bifenthrin or deltamethrin was suggested as insufficient to control *B. tabaci* culture due to its small size. Notwithstanding, according to Arthurs et al. [19], nettings of large mesh size treated with deltamethrin proved insufficient to protect a greenhouse crop from *F. occidentalis* invasion. Hence, both the effect of LLINs on beneficial enemies and their effectiveness in small sized insects should be further evaluated [18].

Recently, Rumbos et al. [17] successfully demonstrated the efficacy of Carifend®, a polyester net coated with alpha-cypermethrin, against two stored tobacco insect pests, the cigarette beetle, *Lasioderma serricorne* (F.) (Coleoptera: Anobiidae) and the tobacco moth, *Ephestia elutella* (Hübner) (Lepidoptera: Pyralidae). Moreover, Paloukas et al. [20] suggested that Carifend® could be effectively used to control different major stored-product insects such as the rice weevil, *Sitophilus oryzae* (L.) (Coleoptera: Curculionidae), since 98% mortality was recorded two weeks after the exposure to the treated net.

The use of nanoparticles as a novel biological insect control agent has been well established in the recent years. Silicon is known as the most frequent metalloid and the most copious element on earth after oxygen [21–23]. The mode of action of silicon dioxide (SiO_2) begins with the adherence of the nanoparticles on the cuticle of the insect, inactivating epicuticular lipids, which leads to death through desiccation [24,25]. Furthermore, Rastogi et al. [22], suggested that the mortality of pests could be related to congestion of spiracles and tracheas caused by the nanosilica particles.

Diatomaceous earth (DE) that consists mainly of amorphous hydrated silica has been extensively used in stored product insect management. Vayias and Athanassiou [26] stated that the effectiveness of DE is associated with the developmental stage of the insects. Indeed, the management of the confused flour beetle adults, *Tribolium confusum* Jacquelin DuVal (Coleoptera: Tenebrionidae) is considerably difficult compared to soft-bodied greenhouse pests such as aphids. On the other hand, aphids are among the most common pests in horticultural crops and are related to the transmission of many economically hazardous viruses even after injecting their sucking mouthparts on the leaves for a very short time interval [18,27]. Unlike hard-bodied beetles, aphids are considered to be much more vulnerable to desiccation from sorptive materials and micro-wounds. For instance, Singh and Singh [28] found that DEs could cause rapid mortality of the aphid *Rhopalosiphum padi* (L.) (Homoptera: Aphididae), when applied on wheat plants. However, in that study, the authors stood eventually against these DE applications, because of negative photosynthetic rates [28].

Recently, Shoaib et al. [29], indicated that the exposure of larvae of *Plutella xylostella* (L.) (Lepidoptera: Plutellidae) to 1 mg × cm^{-2} of a siliceous dust formulation resulted in 85% mortality after 72 h. The authors suggested that the mortality rate is improved as dose and exposure interval are increased. Moreover, silica nanoparticles, concerning their physical and chemical properties, differ significantly from their bulk formation [19]. According to Debnath et al. [30], nanoparticles proved to be much more effective when compared with bulk silica against *S. oryzae*. At the post-harvest stages of agricultural commodities, stored product protection could be enhanced by the use of silicon-based nanoparticles as non-conventional pesticide agents [2,31].

To date, little attention has been given to the incorporation of physical inert dusts to the yarns of insect proof nets. The application of non-toxic and environmental-friendly nets could replace the insecticidal treated nets leading to insecticide-free products. Thus, the objective of our study was to assess the effectiveness of silicon dioxide-treated nets under laboratory conditions for the control of the black bean aphid, *Aphis fabae* Scopoli (Hemipetra: Aphididae), and the stored product pests *T. confusum* and *S. oryzae*. The aforementioned species were exposed to insect proof nets coated with two different silicon dioxide dust formulations, Syloid®ED3 and Syloid®ED5 with and without the addition of paraffin in order to achieve better particle adherence to the net, respectively.

2. Materials and Methods

2.1. Insects Tested

The rearing of the *A. fabae* individuals took place at the Laboratory of Agricultural Entomology, Benaki Phytopathological Institute, Attica, Greece. Aphids were reared on *Vicia faba* L. plants at 20 ± 1 °C, relative humidity (r.h.) of 65 ± 2% and a photoperiod of 16 h in light: 8 h in dark [32]. Aphid colonies were transferred to the Laboratory of Entomology and Agricultural Zoology (LEAZ), Department of Agriculture, Crop Production and Rural Environment, University of Thessaly to carry out the bioassays.

Established laboratory colonies of *S. oryzae* and *T. confusum* were maintained in LEAZ under controlled conditions in a growth chamber as suggested by Faliagka et al. [33].

2.2. Nettings and Dust Formulations

Experiments were carried out with four samples of the same insect proof net, the textiles of which were performed by the Institut für Textiltechnik (ITA) of RWTH Aachen University. The weaving and the evaluation of the nets was provided from Thrace Nonwovens & Geosynthetics S.A. (Thrace, Greece). All textiles were coated either with Syloid® ED3 or Syloid® ED5 which are amorphous silica dust formulations (P&S Powder and Surface GmbH, Salzkotten, Germany). The former silica dust consists of 99–100% SiO_2 with particle size of 5.8 µm, while the latter consists of 95–100% SiO_2 with particle size of 9.0 µm. Paraffin was added as an organic primer in two of the four netting samples (ED3-P and ED5-P) consisting of different silica formulation in order to enhance the adhesion properties of each dust to the net. ED3 and ED5 samples were used without the addition of paraffin. The purpose of the primer is the integration of up to 40% more SiO_2 particles on the net. The mass of the deposited silica particles on the net's surface was fluctuated from 0.4 to 0.9 $g \times m^{-2}$ depending on the dust formulation as well as the addition of paraffin. However, paraffin may reduce the mesh size and therefore, the air permeability properties of the tested nets. In the present study, the insecticidal properties of SiO_2 nanoparticles were evaluated. In the case where adequate results are provided, it is suggested to incorporate silica on nets of larger pores in order to alleviate insufficient ventilation. Table 1 shows the properties of the nets used in the experimental trials.

Table 1. Properties of the silicon coated nets ED3 (without paraffin), ED3-P (paraffin), ED5 (without paraffin), and ED5-P (paraffin).

Sample	Mesh Size	Silica Particles Diameter (µm)	Coating Repetition	Mass of Deposited Silica Particles on the Surface of the Net ($g \times m^{-2}$)
ED3	50 mesh	5.8	2	0.4
ED3-P	50 mesh	5.8	2	0.7
ED5	50 mesh	9.0	2	0.7
ED5-P	50 mesh	9.0	2	0.9

All samples were produced by the same 50 mesh net that was constructed by using high density polyethylene (HDPE) monofilament yarns. SiO_2 free-nettings with the same mesh size as well as clear Petri dishes without the addition of nets were used as a control treatment. The silica coating procedure was repeated two times for each tested net.

2.3. Bioassay Series

Nets were fine cut and adjusted at the bottom of plastic Petri dishes (59.4 cm^2 in surface), using a thin layer of silicon. The lids of plastic dishes are usually loose-fitting making it easy for insects to escape, so, the "neck" of each Petri dish was covered with polytetrafluoroethylene dispersion, (Northern Product, Cumberland, RI, USA). A single fine brush was used to insert the species into the Petri dishes to avoid wounding.

2.3.1. Short-Term Effect

In the short-term effect bioassay series, adults of *A. fabae* and *S. oryzae*, and larvae of *T. confusum* were used. Ten insects of each species were transferred to the Petri dishes. All species were exposed to silica-treated nets, clear Petri dishes (without nets), and untreated nets for the intervals of 5, 10, 15, 20, 25, 30, 60, 90, and 180 min. For each exposure interval, mortality and knockdown effect of all species in each Petri dish were recorded. For each of the four nets, the bioassay was replicated eight times per exposure interval. Thus, in this series of bioassays 144 Petri dishes were used in total.

2.3.2. Long-Term Effect

The purpose of this series of bioassays was to evaluate the effect of the nets on the knockdown and mortality rates of the exposed individuals at certain post-exposure intervals. Thus, as above, ten individuals of each species were transferred to Petri dishes, with different plates per species, and exposed to the nets for 15, 30, and 60 min. Knockdown and mortality were recorded immediately after the completion of the exposure periods and then all insects were carefully transferred to new dishes consisting of untreated nets or clear Petri dishes (without nets). When transferring the insects, a clean single fine brush was used to avoid possible contamination of the dust in the treated nets. Within each exposure interval of 15, 30, and 60 min no food was added in the Petri dishes. However, during post-exposure period for *S. oryzae* and *T. confusum*, cracked wheat (0.5 ± 0.1 gr) and wheat flour (1.0 ± 0.1 gr) were added in all petri dishes, respectively. In the case of *A. fabae* no food was supplied, since the bioassay lasted one day, unlike that of the stored product insects which was completed after 10 days. All bioassays were carried out at 25 °C and 65% r.h. Mortality and knockdown effect of *S. oryzae* and *T. confusum* were assessed after 1, 7, and 10 days, whereas in the case of *A. fabae* after 1 day. For each of the four nets, the bioassays were replicated eight times. A total of 624 Petri dishes were used to perform this series of bioassays.

2.4. Statistical Analysis

The results of the first series of bioassay (short-term effect) were analyzed using Probit Analysis to estimate the knockdown time, i.e., KD_{t50}, KD_{t95}, and KD_{t99} for each species and net formulation. The intervals tested yielded a variety of knockdown results only for *A. fabae*, which allowed the calculation of KD_{t50}, KD_{t95}, and KD_{t99} values. For the second series of bioassays, separately of each species, the data (knockdown and mortality) were converted to percentages and then were submitted to a two-way ANOVA, to determine the differences among the exposure intervals (15, 30, and 60 min) and among the net formulations (including controls as well), while means of knockdown and mortality were separated using the Tukey-Kramer HSD test at the 5% level. Moreover, the same approach was conducted for the long-term effect for each species tested. The data were analyzed using SPSS 25.0 (SPSS Inc., Chicago, IL, USA).

3. Results

3.1. Short-Term Effect

The mortality rate of all tested species was relatively low. In the first series of tests, KD_t values were not found to fit the data well, since P values were <0.01 (Table 2). In most of the cases, confidence interval could not be estimated for *A. fabae* and *S. oryzae*, except for ED5-P of *A. fabae*. For *T. confusum*, Probit could not be estimated, since the percentage of knocked down individuals was negligible (data not presented).

Overall, KD_{t99} values for *A. fabae* at ED3-P resulted in the highest values among treatments, corresponding to 1590.9 min (approximately 26 h) (Table 2). Contrariwise, the lowest KD_{t99} value was recorded at ED5-P, corresponding to 363.3 min (approximately 6 h) (Table 2). Moreover, for *S. oryzae* the resulting values were similar with those of *A. fabae* at ED3, which were 1235.7 min (approximately 20 h) and 1281.4 min (approximately 21 h), respectively. For KD_{t50} the lowest value (51.3 min) for *A. fabae* was recorded at ED5, whereas the highest value (279.7 min) was noted at ED3-P (Table 2).

Table 2. Probit analysis for KD_{t50}, KD_{t95}, and KD_{T99} (confidence intervals) of *Aphis fabae* and *Sitophilus oryzae* adults exposed to four different nets (ED3, ED3-P, ED5, ED5-P) for 180 min, values are expressed as minutes to knockdown.

#	Nets	KD_{t50}	KD_{t95}	KD_{t99}	Slope ± SE	χ^2	P
A. fabae	ED3	253.3 [a]	980.2 [a]	1281.4 [a]	2.7 ± 0.1	389.8	<0.01
	ED3-P	279.7 [a]	1206.8 [a]	1590.9 [a]	2.1 ± 0.1	290.9	<0.01
	ED5	51.3 [a]	669.6 [a]	925.8 [a]	3.3 ± 0.1	561.7	<0.01
	ED5-P	74.9 (49.8—109.1)	278.8 (206.6—465.8)	363.3 (265.6—619.5)	9.6 ± 0.1	372.8	<0.01
#	Nets	KD_{t50}	KD_{t95}	KD_{t99}	Slope ± SE	χ^2	P
S. oryzae	ED3	-	-	-	-	-	-
	ED3-P	767.3 [a]	1098.5 [a]	1235.7 [a]	0.6 ± 0.1	449.7	<0.01
	ED5	-	-	-	-	-	-
	ED5-P	-	-	-	-	-	-

[a] Could not estimate confidence intervals; - Could not estimate knockdown time.

3.2. Long-Term Effect

The mortality rate ranged significantly between the tested cases (Tables 3–5). Knockdown of *A. fabae* was low and did not exceed 28.7% (Table 3), whereas mortality was negligible (data not presented). For knocked down individuals, significant differences were noted in all tested net formulations among the time intervals (15, 30, and 60 min). Finally, at the 1-day post-exposure period, mortality was 100% in all tested net formulations (Table 3).

Regarding *S. oryzae* individuals, knockdown and mortality were negligible, in all tested net formulations for the 15, 30, and 60 min intervals (data not presented), while at the 1-day post-exposure period, no significant differences were noted among the exposure intervals (Table 4). At this interval, mortality was generally low, reaching 6.2%. However, in most of the cases, at the 7-day post-exposure period mortality was approximately 87%, even when the initial exposure was 15 min, while after 10 days mortality reached 100% (Table 4).

Regarding *T. confusum* larvae, knockdown and mortality were generally low (<5%, data not presented). Larval knockdown of *T. confusum* was also negligible (data not presented). After 7 d of exposure in all formulations, mortality did not exceed 30%, whereas after 10 d the highest mortality level was 34% at ED5-P (Table 5). Significant differences were recorded among the exposure intervals in most of the cases (Table 5).

Table 3. Short- and long-term knockdown (KD) and mortality (% ± SE) of *Aphis fabae* adults exposed for 15, 30, and 60 min to dishes with four different treated nets (ED3, ED3-P, ED5, ED5-P), dishes with untreated net and dishes without net. The first day after exposure for each exposure interval is considered as the long-term effect.

Exposure time	ED3				ED3-P				ED5				ED5-P				Untreated net				Without net			
	Short term		Long term		Short term		Long term		Short term		Long term		Short term		Long term		Short term		Long term		Short term		Long term	
	KD	Mortality	KD	Mortality	KD	Mortality	KD	Mortality	KD	Mortality	KD	Mortality	KD	Mortality	KD	Mortality	KD	Mortality	KD	Mortality	KD	Mortality	KD	Mortality
15 min	0.0 ± 0.0 a		0.0 ± 0.0 A	100.0 ± 0.0 A	0.0 ± 0.0 a		0.0 ± 0.0 A	100.0 ± 0.0 A	0.0 ± 0.0 a		0.0 ± 0.0 A	100.0 ± 0.0 A	0.0 ± 0.0 a		0.0 ± 0.0 A	100.0 ± 0.0 A	0.0 ± 0.0		2.5 ± 2.5 A		0.0 ± 0.0		20.0 ± 3.2 B	36.2 ± 8.6 B
30 min	0.0 ± 0.0 a		5.0 ± 1.8 A	100.0 ± 0.0 A	0.0 ± 0.0 a		0.0 ± 0.0 A	100.0 ± 0.0 A	0.0 ± 0.0 a		0.0 ± 0.0 A	100.0 ± 0.0 A	0.0 ± 0.0 a		0.0 ± 0.0 A	100.0 ± 0.0 A	0.0 ± 0.0		0.0 ± 0.0 A		0.0 ± 0.0		22.5 ± 13.1 B	12.5 ± 3.1 B
60 min	27.5 ± 4.5 bA	22.5 ± 3.1 bA	98.7 ± 1.2 A	100.0 ± 0.0 A	28.7 ± 3.9 bA	22.5 ± 3.1 bA	0.0 ± 0.0 A	100.0 ± 0.0 A	0.0 ± 0.0 a	0.0 ± 0.0 A	0.0 ± 0.0 A	100.0 ± 0.0 A	15.0 ± 4.6 bA	0.0 ± 0.0 A	0.0 ± 0.0 A	93.7 ± 4.1 A	0.0 ± 0.0 B	0.0 ± 0.0 B	0.0 ± 0.0 B		0.0 ± 0.0 B		16.2 ± 4.6 B	23.7 ± 6.7 B
F	36.8	51.5	0.6	1.0	52.1		0.7	1.0					10.5			2.2			1.0				0.1	3.2
P	<0.01	<0.01	0.55	0.38	<0.01		0.50	0.38					<0.01			0.13			0.38				0.86	0.06

Within each exposure time, post-exposure interval, and net formulation, means followed by the same lowercase letters (a, b) do not differ significantly according to Tukey-Kramer HSD test at P < 0.05. Within each exposure interval, post-exposure interval, and net formulation, mortality, and knockdown means followed by the same uppercase letters (A, B) do not differ significantly across treatments according to Tukey-Kramer HSD test at P < 0.05. Where no letter exist, no significant differences were noted. ANOVA parameters for long-term effect and knocked down adults were: at 15 min F = 22.8, P < 0.01, 30 min, F = 2.9, P = 0.02, 60 min, F = 12.4, P < 0.01, whereas for short-term effect and knocked down adults at 60 min, F = 22.9, P < 0.01. For delayed mortality at 15 min, F = 54.3, P < 0.01, 30 min, F = 779.5, P < 0.01, 60 min, F = 88.7, P < 0.01, in all cases df = 2, 23. In the case where "-" is indicated, F and P values were not provided in the Table since no variances among the samples were recorded.

Table 4. Delayed mortality (% ± SE) of *Sitophilus oryzae* adults exposed for 15, 30, and 60 min to dishes with four different nets (ED3, ED3-P, ED5, ED5-P), dishes with untreated net and dishes without net. The 1st, 7th and 10th day after exposure for each exposure interval is considered as the long-term effect.

Exposure time (d)	ED3			ED3-P			ED5			ED5-P			Untreated Net			Without Net		
	1st	7th	10th	1st	7th	10th	1st	7th	10th	1st	7th	10th	1st	7th	10th	1st	7th	10th
15 min	2.5 ± 1.6	100.0 ± 0.0 A	100.0 ± 0.0 A	0.0 ± 0.0	97.5 ± 2.5 A	98.7 ± 1.2 A	0.0 ± 0.0	100.0 ± 0.0 aA	100.0 ± 0.0 aA	5.0 ± 1.8	100.0 ± 0.0 bA	100.0 ± 0.0 aA	6.2 ± 4.1	40.0 ± 8.4 B	56.2 ± 9.0 B	0.0 ± 0.0	0.0 ± 0.0 C	11.2 ± 2.2 C
30 min	3.7 ± 1.8	97.5 ± 2.5 A	100.0 ± 0.0 A	5.0 ± 1.8	97.5 ± 1.6 A	100.0 ± 0.0 A	0.0 ± 0.0	96.2 ± 1.8 bA	96.2 ± 1.8 bA	3.7 ± 2.6	97.5 ± 2.5 abA	100.0 ± 0.0 aA	2.5 ± 1.6	22.5 ± 10.6 B	30.0 ± 11.0 B	0.0 ± 0.0	0.0 ± 0.0 C	11.2 ± 2.9 C
60 min	2.5 ± 1.6	98.7 ± 1.2 A	100.0 ± 0.0 A	3.7 ± 1.8	100.0 ± 0.0 A	100.0 ± 0.0 A	0.0 ± 0.0	100.0 ± 0.0 aA	100.0 ± 0.0 aA	0.0 ± 0.0	87.5 ± 5.2 aA	88.7 ± 5.4 bA	2.5 ± 2.5	43.7 ± 9.9 B	56.2 ± 9.8 B	0.0 ± 0.0	0.0 ± 0.0 C	12.5 ± 3.1 C
F	0.8	0.6		2.9	1.0	1.0		4.2	4.2	1.9	3.9	4.2	0.5	1.3	2.3			0.1
P	0.83	0.55		0.07	0.38	0.38		0.02	0.02	0.16	0.03	0.02	0.59	0.27	0.12			0.93

Within each exposure time, post-exposure interval, and net formulation, means followed by the same lowercase letters (a, b) do not differ significantly according to the Tukey-Kramer HSD test at P < 0.05. Within each exposure interval, post-exposure interval, and net formulation, mortality means followed by the same uppercase letters (A, B) do not differ significantly across treatments according to the Tukey-Kramer HSD test at P < 0.05. Where no letters exist, no significant differences were noted. ANOVA parameters for 1st day were: at 15 min, F = 1.9, P = 0.10, 30 min, F = 1.6, P = 0.18, 60 min, F = 1.3, P = 0.26, for 7th day were: at 15 min, F = 142.2, P < 0.01, 30 min, F = 91.9, P < 0.01, 60 min, F = 79.1, P < 0.01, whereas for 10th day were: at 15 min, F = 92.2, P < 0.01, 30 min, F = 75.4, P < 0.01, 60 min, F = 55.6, P < 0.01, in all cases df = 5, 47. In the case where "-" is indicated, F and P values were not provided in the Table since no variances among the samples were recorded.

Table 5. Delayed mortality (% ± SE) of *Tribolium confusum* larvae exposed for 15, 30, and 60 min to dishes with four different nets (ED3, ED3-P, ED5, ED5-P), dishes with untreated net and dishes without net. The 1st, 7th, and 10th day after exposure for each exposure interval is considered as the long-term effect.

Exposure time (d)	ED3			ED3-P			ED5			ED5-P			Untreated net			Without Net		
	1st	7th	10th	1st	7th	10th	1st	7th	10th	1st	7th	10th	1st	7th	10th	1st	7th	10th
15 min	3.7 ± 2.6	12.5 ± 3.1 ab	13.7 ± 3.2	1.2 ± 1.2 a	8.7 ± 4.4 a	18.7 ± 3.5	2.5 ± 1.6 ab	13.7 ± 4.1	28.7 ± 2.9 a	2.5 ± 1.6	11.2 ± 4.7 ab	18.7 ± 5.4 ab	6.2 ± 2.6	5.0 ± 1.8	16.2 ± 3.7	0.0 ± 0.0	3.7 ± 2.6	28.7 ± 5.1
30 min	0.0 ± 0.0	7.5 ± 2.5 aA	12.5 ± 3.6	2.5 ± 1.6 ab	18.7 ± 3.5 abB	20.0 ± 3.7	0.0 ± 0.0 a	6.2 ± 2.6 A	8.7 ± 2.2 b	0.0 ± 0.0	8.7 ± 2.2 aAB	11.2 ± 1.2 a	2.5 ± 2.5	7.5 ± 2.5 A	18.7 ± 6.3	0.0 ± 0.0	12.2 ± 1.2 A	21.2 ± 3.5
60 min	6.2 ± 1.8 B	20.0 ± 4.2 bAB	22.5 ± 3.6	7.5 ± 1.6 bB	30.0 ± 5.3 bB	32.5 ± 5.2	7.5 ± 2.5 bB	16.2 ± 3.7 AB	25.0 ± 3.7 a	3.7 ± 1.8 AB	26.5 ± 6.5 bB	33.7 ± 7.0 b	3.7 ± 1.8 AB	6.2 ± 3.2 A	15.0 ± 4.2	0.0 ± 0.0 A	2.5 ± 1.6 A	22.5 ± 3.1
F	2.9	3.5	2.4	4.7	5.6	3.2	4.9	2.1	12.0	1.8	3.8	4.8	0.7	0.2	0.1	-	0.4	1.0
P	0.07	0.04	0.11	0.02	0.01	0.06	0.01	0.14	0.01	0.18	0.03	0.01	0.52	0.79	0.86	-	0.66	0.38

Within each exposure interval, post-exposure interval, and net formulation mortality, means followed by the same lowercase letter do not differ significantly according to the Tukey-Kramer HSD test at $P < 0.05$. Within each exposure interval, post-exposure interval, and net formulation, mortality means followed by the same uppercase letter do not differ significantly across treatments according to the Tukey-Kramer HSD test at $P < 0.05$. Where no letters exist, no significant differences were noted. ANOVA parameters for 1st day were: at 15 min, F = 1.3, P = 0.6, 30 min, F = 1.1, P = 0.36, 60 min, F = 2.6, P = 0.03, for 7th day were: at 15 min, F = 1.2, P = 0.30, 30 min, F = 5.1, P < 0.01, 60 min, F = 6.1, P < 0.01, whereas for 10th day were: at 15 min, F = 2.4, P = 0.05, 30 min, F = 1.9, P = 0.12, 60min, F = 2.2, P = 0.07, in all cases $df = 5, 47$. In the case where "-" is indicated, F and P values were not provided in the Table since no variances among the samples were recorded.

4. Discussion

The results of our study indicated that even in the case of the longest exposure interval (180 min) no immediate mortality was achieved for either of the stored product species tested. However, for *A. fabae*, knockdown effect was vigorous and rapid, especially at longer intervals, as KD_{t50} was high after approximately one hour. In general, from the most to the least susceptible, the species/life stages tested here can be classified as *A. fabae* adults > *S. oryzae* adults > *T. confusum* larvae.

Particle size is highly associated with the insecticidal efficacy of inert dusts. Many authors have emphasized on the importance of the particle size, a significant physical property of dust formulations, underlining that formulations of smaller particles may enhance the insecticidal efficacy on a variety of stored-product beetles [34–39]. Korunić [40] found that the efficacy of DEs is promoted when particle size ranges between 1 and 30 μm. Similarly, Vayias et al. [38] indicated that DEs particles, sized up to 45 μm, resulted in higher mortality of stored product beetles, as compared with larger particles. However, Korunić [40] underlined the significance of the DEs origin, and concluded that even a high range between the size of particles (i.e., 0–192 μm) could lead to similar insecticidal results, indicating the significance of the particle shape. In this context, Rumbos et al. [39] found that the insecticidal effect of zeolites on the control of stored-product pests was not highly associated with particle size.

Peng et al. [41] stated that the dispersity and stability of SiO_2 nanoparticles are enhanced when added to liquid paraffin. In the present study, it was concluded that the susceptibility of *A. fabae* and *S. oryzae* was high, regardless of the addition of the primer or the size of silica nanoparticles, since no significant differences were recorded concerning the long-term effect. Notwithstanding, our results suggested that the use of paraffin on the net's surface contributes to the reduction of fabrics' shrinkage whereas it increases the rate of the particle deposition. Thus, the knockdown effect of *A. fabae* was increased when insects were exposed to ED5-P nets since in this case, the deposition of silica particles was the highest among all tested samples due to the addition of paraffin. In particular, it was shown that 99% of the adults were knocked down after six hours when exposed to the net coated with the ED5-P dust formulation, which consisted of the largest silica particles at the highest deposition rate.

Silica particles should not be considered as the only lethal factor in our study, as mortality can be also attributed to the presence of the net itself. As shown in the results corresponding to the control treatments, insects exposed to the SiO_2-free nets were also affected by the presence of the net as opposed to the insects exposed to the dishes without net. Concerning the above, silica-treated nets could be applied on the vent openings of a greenhouse limiting the number of infestations due to greenhouse pests' invasions, which occurs mechanically, i.e., without the use of the dust. A similar approach has been investigated in the case of stored product insects, with similar results regarding the detrimental effect of the net to the insect bodies [17,20].

Although no immediate mortality was recorded for all the insect species tested, delayed mortality was high, reaching 100% even in the shortest exposure time (15 min). Similarly, Kavallieratos et al. [42] observed a significant delayed mortality on 14 d for *S. oryzae* and the lesser grain borer, *Rhyzopertha dominica* (F.) (Coleoptrea: Bostrychidae) when exposed to a mixture of DE and abamectin. Our data show that, despite low initial effect, delayed mortality for the two beetle species was high, which clearly suggests that the exposed individuals were heavily affected by the presence of the dusts in their cuticles. As inert materials are slow-acting, it has been observed that mortality may take several days or even weeks to occur, even if the insects are in continuous contact with the dust particles [43,44]. Nevertheless, the current results suggest that even the shortest exposure to the dust particles tested here is irreversibly lethal, and recovery is less likely to appear. This is particularly important, as insects will eventually die after their removal from the treated substrate, a characteristic that is even more important in the case of aphids, if it is combined with the knockdown that appears rapidly after exposure.

To conclude, this study indicates that all of the nets tested here were effective for the control of aphids and less for beetles (including larval stage), despite variations in efficacy among treatments. Practically, the nets that are coated with inert materials can serve as a good alternatives to traditional pesticides in greenhouses but also in food and processing facilities, significantly moderating insect immigration. This technology can be adopted in a wide range of facilities, and also in food packaging, where the larval stage can penetrate with ease. At the same time, in a "real world" greenhouse scenario, immigration of aphids from the outside toward the plantation will force the insects to pass through the treated net, which is expected to be lethal, even if some aphids eventually pass successfully.

Author Contributions: Conceptualization, N.K., M.O., P.A. and C.G.A.; methodology, P.A., S.F. and E.L.; formal analysis, E.L., P.A. and S.F.; investigation, P.A., S.F., E.L., N.K. and C.G.A.; resources, N.K., C.G.A.; writing—original draft preparation, P.A., S.F., E.L., C.G.A. and N.K.; writing—review and editing, P.A., S.F., E.L., C.G.A. and N.K.; visualization, N.K., M.P. and M.O.; supervision, C.G.A. and N.K.; project administration, N.K., M.O. and M.P.; funding acquisition, N.K. and C.G.A. All authors have read and agreed to the published version of the manuscript.

Funding: This research has been co-financed by the European Union and Greek national funds through the National Action "Bilateral and Multilateral E&T Cooperation Greece-Germany" (project code: T2DGE-0120). Furthermore, this research has been co-financed by the European Union and Greek national funds through the Operational Program Competitiveness, Entrepreneurship and Innovation, under the call RESEARCH—CREATE—INNOVATE (project code:T1EDK-01491).

Acknowledgments: This research has been co-financed by the European Union and Greek national funds through the National Action "Bilateral and Multilateral E&T Cooperation Greece-Germany" (project code: T2DGE-0120). Furthermore, this research has been co-financed by the European Union and Greek national funds through the Operational Program Competitiveness, Entrepreneurship and Innovation, under the call RESEARCH—CREATE—INNOVATE (project code:T1EDK-01491).

Conflicts of Interest: The authors declare no conflict of interest.

References

1. Boyer, S.; Zhang, H.; Lempérière, G. A review of control methods and resistance mechanisms in stored-product insects. *Bull. Entomol. Res.* **2012**, *102*, 213–229. [CrossRef] [PubMed]
2. Athanassiou, C.-G.; Kavallieratos, N.-G.; Benelli, G.; Losic, D.; Usha Rani, P.; Desneux, N. Nanoparticles for pest control: Current status and future perspectives. *J. Pest Sci.* **2017**, *91*, 1–15. [CrossRef]
3. Awolola, T.-S.; Adeogun, A.; Olakiigbe, A.-K.; Oyeniyi, T.; Olukosi, Y.-A.; Okoh, H.; Arowolo, T.; Akila, J.; Oduola, A.; Amajoh, C.-N. Pyrethroids resistance intensity and resistance mechanisms in *Anopheles gambiae* from malaria vector surveillance sites in Nigeria. *PLoS ONE* **2018**, *13*, e0205230. [CrossRef]
4. Aktar, W.; Sengupta, D.; Chowdhury, A. Impact of pesticides use in agriculture: Their benefits and hazards. *Interdiscip. Toxicol.* **2009**, *2*, 1–12. [CrossRef] [PubMed]
5. Mukherjee, A.; Knoch, S.; Chouinard, G.; Tavares, J.-R.; Dumont, M.-J. Use of bio-based polymers in agricultural exclusion nets: A perspective. *Biosyst. Eng.* **2019**, *180*, 121–145. [CrossRef]
6. Kittas, C.; Katsoulas, N.; Bartzanas, T.; Mermier, M.; Boulard, T. The impact of insect screens and ventilation openings on the greenhouse microclimate. *Trans. ASABE* **2008**, *51*, 2151–2165. [CrossRef]
7. Kitta, E.; Baille, A.-D.; Katsoulas, N.; Rigakis, N.; González-Real, M.-M. Effects of cover optical properties on screenhouse radiative environment and sweet pepper productivity. *Biosyst. Eng.* **2014**, *122*, 115–126. [CrossRef]
8. Teitel, M. The effect of screened openings on greenhouse microclimate. *Agric. For. Meteorol.* **2007**, *143*, 159–175. [CrossRef]
9. Dáder, B.; Legarrea, S.; Moreno, A.; Ambros, C.-M.; Fereres, A.; Skovmand, O.; Bosselmann, R.; Viñuela, E. Insecticide-treated nets as a new approach to control vegetable pests in protected crops. *Acta Hortic.* **2014**, *1015*, 103–112. [CrossRef]
10. Rigakis, N.; Katsoulas, N.; Teitel, M.; Bartzanas, T.; Kittas, C. A simple model for ventilation rate determination in screenhouses. *Energy Build.* **2015**, *87*, 293–301. [CrossRef]
11. Bell, M.-L.; Baker, J.-R. Comparison of greenhouse screening materials for excluding whitefly (Homoptera: Aleyrodidae) and thrips (Thysanoptera: Thripidae). *J. Econ. Entomol.* **2000**, *93*, 800–804. [CrossRef] [PubMed]
12. Parra, J.-P.; Baeza, E.; Montero, J.-I.; Bailey, B.-J. Natural ventilation of parral greenhouses. *Biosyst. Eng.* **2004**, *87*, 355–366. [CrossRef]
13. Fatnassi, H.; Boulard, T.; Demrati, H.; Bouirden, L.; Sappe, G. Ventilation performance of a large Canarian-type greenhouse equipped with insect-proof nets. *Biosyst. Eng.* **2002**, *82*, 97–105. [CrossRef]
14. Katsoulas, N.; Bartzanas, T.; Boulard, T.; Mermier, M.; Kittas, C. Effect of vent openings and insect screens on greenhouse ventilation. *Biosyst. Eng.* **2006**, *93*, 427–436. [CrossRef]

15. Baeza, E.-J.; Pérez-Parra, J.-J.; Montero, J.-I.; Bailey, B.-J.; López, J.-C.; Gázquez, J.-C. Analysis of the role of sidewall vents on buoyancy-driven natural ventilation in parral-type greenhouses with and without insect screens using computational fluid dynamics. *Biosyst. Eng.* **2009**, *104*, 86–96. [CrossRef]
16. Chouinard, G.; Veilleux, J.; Pelletier, F.; Larose, M.; Philion, V.; Cormier, D. Impact of exclusion netting row covers on arthropod presence and crop damage to 'Honeycrisp' apple trees in North America: A five-year study. *Crop Prot.* **2017**, *98*, 248–254. [CrossRef]
17. Rumbos, C.-I.; Sakka, M.; Schaffert, S.; Sterz, T.; Austin, J.-W.; Bozoglou, C.; Klitsinaris, P.; Athanassiou, C.-G. Evaluation of Carifend®, an alpha-cypermethrin-coated polyester net, for the control of *Lasioderma serricorne* and *Ephestia elutella* in stored tobacco. *J. Pest Sci.* **2018**, *91*, 751–759. [CrossRef]
18. Dáder, B.; Legarrea, S.; Moreno, A.; Plaza, M.; Carmo-Sousa, M.; Amor, F.; Viñuela, E.; Fereres, A. Control of insect vectors and plant viruses in protected crops by novel pyrethroid-treated nets. *Pest Manag. Sci.* **2014**, *71*, 1397–1406. [CrossRef] [PubMed]
19. Arthurs, S.-P.; Krauter, P.-C.; Gilder, K.; Heinz, K.-M. Evaluation of deltamethrin-impregnated nets as a protective barrier against Western flower thrips, *Frankliniella occidentalis* (Thysanoptera: Thripidae) under laboratory and greenhouse conditions. *Crop Prot.* **2018**, *112*, 227–231. [CrossRef]
20. Paloukas, Y.-Z.; Agrafioti, P.; Rumbos, C.-I.; Schaffert, S.; Sterz, T.; Bozoglou, C.; Klitsinaris, P.; Austin, J.-W.; Athanassiou, C.-G. Evaluation of Carifend® for the control of stored-product beetles. *J. Stored Prod. Res.* **2020**, *85*. [CrossRef]
21. Epstein, E. The anomaly of silicon in plant biology. *Proc. Natl. Acad. Sci. USA* **1994**, *91*, 11–17. [CrossRef] [PubMed]
22. Rastogi, A.; Tripathi, D.-K.; Yadav, S.; Chauhan, D.-K.; Živčák, M.; Ghorbanpour, M.; El-Sheery, N.-I.; Brestic, M. Application of silicon nanoparticles in agriculture. *3 Biotech* **2019**, *9*, 90. [CrossRef] [PubMed]
23. Debnath, N.; Mitra, S.; Das, S.; Goswami, A. Synthesis of surface functionalized silica nanoparticles and their use as entomotoxic nanocides. *Powder Technol.* **2012**, *221*, 252–256. [CrossRef]
24. Barik, T.-K.; Sahu, B.; Swain, V. Nanosilica—From medicine to pest control. *Parasitol. Res.* **2008**, *103*, 253–258. [CrossRef]
25. Benelli, G. Mode of action of nanoparticles against insects. *Environ. Sci. Pollut. Res.* **2018**, *25*, 12329–12341. [CrossRef]
26. Vayias, B.-J.; Athanassiou, C.-G. Factors affecting the insecticidal efficacy of the diatomaceous earth formulation SilicoSec against adults and larvae of the confused flour beetle, *Tribolium confusum* DuVal (Coleoptera: Tenebrionidae). *Crop Prot.* **2004**, *23*, 565–573. [CrossRef]
27. Ng, J.C.-K.; Perry, K.-L. Transmission of plant viruses by aphid vectors. *Mol. Plant Pathol.* **2004**, *5*, 505–511. [CrossRef]
28. Singh, B.; Singh, V. Laboratory and field studies demonstrating the insecticidal potential of diatomaceous earth against wheat aphids in rice-wheat cropping system of Punjab (India). *Cereal Res. Commun.* **2016**, *44*, 435–443. [CrossRef]
29. Shoaib, A.; Elabasy, A.; Waqas, M.; Lin, L.; Cheng, X.; Zhang, Q.; Shi, Z.H. Entomotoxic effect of silicon dioxide nanoparticles on *Plutella xylostella* (L.) (Lepidoptera: Plutellidae) under laboratory conditions. *Toxicol. Environ. Chem.* **2018**, *100*, 80–91. [CrossRef]
30. Debnath, N.; Das, S.; Seth, D.; Chandra, R.; Bhattacharya, S.-C.; Goswami, A. Entomotoxic effect of silica nanoparticles against *Sitophilus oryzae* (L.). *J. Pest Sci.* **2011**, *84*, 99–105. [CrossRef]
31. Eroglu, N.; Emekci, M.; Athanassiou, C.-G. Applications of natural zeolites on agriculture and food production. *J. Sci. Food Agric.* **2017**, *97*, 3487–3499. [CrossRef] [PubMed]
32. Papanikolaou, N.-E.; Martinou, A.-F.; Kontodimas, D.-C.; Matsinos, Y.-G.; Milonas, P.-G. Functional responses of immature stages of *Propylea quatuordecimpunctata* (Coleoptera: Coccinellidae) to *Aphis fabae* (Hemiptera: Aphididae). *Eur. J. Entomol.* **2011**, *108*, 391–395. [CrossRef]
33. Faliagka, S.; Agrafioti, P.; Lampiri, E.; Katsoulas, N.; Athanassiou, C.G. Assessment of different inert dust formulations for the control of *Sitophilus oryzae*, *Tribolium confusum* and *Aphis fabae*. *Crop Prot.* **2020**, *137*, 105312. [CrossRef]
34. Kavallieratos, N.-G.; Athanassiou, C.-G.; Vayias, B.-J.; Kotzamanidis, S.; Synodis, S.-D. Efficacy and adherence ratio of diatomaceous earth and spinosad in three wheat varieties against three stored-prosuct insect pests. *J. Stored Prod. Res.* **2010**, *46*, 73–80. [CrossRef]

35. Kavallieratos, N.-G.; Athanassiou, C.-G.; Mpassoukou, A.-E.; Mpakou, F.-D.; Tomanovic, Z.; Manessioti, T.-B.; Papadopoulou, S.-C. Bioassays with diatomaceous earth formulations: Effect of species co-occurrenece, size of vials and application technique. *J. Stored Prod. Res.* **2012**, *42*, 170–179. [CrossRef]
36. Athanassiou, C.-G.; Kavallieratos, N.-G.; Andris, N.-S. Insecticide effect of three diatomaceous earth formulations against adults of *Sitophlus oryzae* (Coleoptera: Curcilionidae) and *Tribolium confusum* (Coleoptera: Tenebrionidae) on oat, rye and triticale. *J. Econ. Entomol.* **2004**, *97*, 2160–2167. [CrossRef]
37. Athanassiou, C.-G.; Vassilakos, N.-T.; Dutton, A.-C.; Jeesop, N.; Sherwood, D.; Pease, G.; Brglez, A.; Storm, C.; Trdan, S. Combining electrostatic powder with an insecticide: Effect on stored prosuct beetles and on the commodity. *Pest Manag. Sci.* **2016**, *72*, 2208–2217. [CrossRef]
38. Vayias, B.-J.; Athanassiou, C.-G.; Korunic, Z.; Rozman, V. Evaluation of natural diatomaceous earth deposits from south-eastern Europe for stored-grain protection: The effect of particle size. *Pest Manag. Sci.* **2009**, *65*, 1118–1123. [CrossRef]
39. Rumbos, C.-I.; Sakka, M.; Berillis, P.; Athanassiou, C.-G. Insecticidal potential of zeolite formulations against three stored-grain insects, particle size effect, adherence to kernels and influence on test weight of grains. *J. Stored Prod. Res.* **2016**, *68*, 93–101. [CrossRef]
40. Korunić, Z. Rapid assessment of the insecticidal value of diatomaceous earths without conducting bioassays. *J. Stored Prod. Res.* **1997**, *33*, 219–229. [CrossRef]
41. Peng, D.-X.; Kang, Y.; Hwang, R.-M.; Shyr, S.-S.; Chang, Y.-P. Tribological properties of diamond and SiO_2 nanoparticles added in paraffin. *Tribol. Int.* **2009**, *42*, 911–917. [CrossRef]
42. Kavallieratos, N.-G.; Athanassiou, C.-G.; Korunic, Z.; Mikeli, N.-H. Evaluations of three novel diatomaceous earths against three stored-grain beetle species on wheat and maize. *Crop Prot.* **2015**, *75*, 132–138. [CrossRef]
43. Subramanyam, B.; Roesli, R. Inert dusts. In *Alternatives to Pesticides in Stored-Product IPM*; Springer: Boston, MA, USA, 2000; pp. 321–380.
44. Athanassiou, C.-G.; Vayias, B.-J.; Dimizas, C.-B.; Kavallieratos, N.-G.; Papagregoriou, A.-S.; Buchelos, C.-T. Insecticidal efficacy of diatomaceous earth against *Sitophilus oryzae* (L.) (Coleoptera: Curculionidae) and *Tribolium confusum* du Val (Coleoptera: Tenebrionidae) on stored wheat: Influence of dose rate, temperature and exposure interval. *J. Stored Prod. Res.* **2005**, *41*, 47–55. [CrossRef]

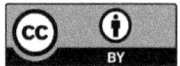

© 2020 by the authors. Licensee MDPI, Basel, Switzerland. This article is an open access article distributed under the terms and conditions of the Creative Commons Attribution (CC BY) license (http://creativecommons.org/licenses/by/4.0/).

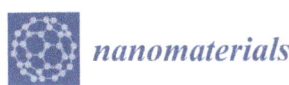

Article

Developing a Highly Stable *Carlina acaulis* Essential Oil Nanoemulsion for Managing *Lobesia botrana*

Giovanni Benelli [1,*], Lucia Pavoni [2], Valeria Zeni [1], Renato Ricciardi [1], Francesca Cosci [1], Gloria Cacopardo [1], Saverio Gendusa [2], Eleonora Spinozzi [2], Riccardo Petrelli [2], Loredana Cappellacci [2], Filippo Maggi [2], Roman Pavela [3,4], Giulia Bonacucina [2] and Andrea Lucchi [1]

[1] Department of Agriculture, Food and Environment, University of Pisa, via del Borghetto 80, 56124 Pisa, Italy; valeriazeni93@gmail.com (V.Z.); renato_ricciardi@hotmail.it (R.R.); francesca.cosci1@virgilio.it (F.C.); gloria.cacopardo@hotmail.com (G.C.); andrea.lucchi@unipi.it (A.L.)
[2] School of Pharmacy, University of Camerino, 62032 Camerino, Italy; lucia.pavoni@unicam.it (L.P.); saverio.gendusa@studenti.unicam.it (S.G.); eleonora.spinozzi@unicam.it (E.S.); riccardo.petrelli@unicam.it (R.P.); loredana.cappellacci@unicam.it (L.C.); filippo.maggi@unicam.it (F.M.); giulia.bonacucina@unicam.it (G.B.)
[3] Crop Research Institute, Drnovska 507, 161 06 Prague, Czech Republic; pavela@vurv.cz
[4] Department of Plant Protection, Czech University of Life Sciences Prague, Kamycka 129, 165 00 Praha 6, Suchdol, Czech Republic
* Correspondence: giovanni.benelli@unipi.it; Tel.: +39-0502216141

Received: 20 July 2020; Accepted: 15 September 2020; Published: 18 September 2020

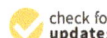

Abstract: The growing interest in the development of green pest management strategies is leading to the exploitation of essential oils (EOs) as promising botanical pesticides. In this respect, nanotechnology could efficiently support the use of EOs through their encapsulation into stable nanoformulations, such as nanoemulsions (NEs), to improve their stability and efficacy. This technology assures the improvement of the chemical stability, hydrophilicity, and environmental persistence of EOs, giving an added value for the fabrication of natural insecticides effective against a wide spectrum of insect vectors and pests of public and agronomical importance. *Carlina acaulis* (Asteraceae) root EO has been recently proposed as a promising ingredient of a new generation of botanical insecticides. In the present study, a highly stable *C. acaulis*-based NE was developed. Interestingly, such a nanosystem was able to encapsulate 6% (*w*/*w*) of *C. acaulis* EO, showing a mean diameter of around 140 nm and a SOR (surfactant-to-oil ratio) of 0.6. Its stability was evaluated in a storage period of six months and corroborated by an accelerated stability study. Therefore, the *C. acaulis* EO and *C. acaulis*-based NE were evaluated for their toxicity against 1st instar larvae of the European grapevine moth (EGVM), *Lobesia botrana* (Denis & Schiffermüller, 1775) (Lepidoptera: Tortricidae), a major vineyard pest. The chemical composition of *C. acaulis* EO was investigated by gas chromatography–mass spectrometry (GC–MS) revealing carlina oxide, a polyacetylene, as the main constituent. In toxicity assays, both the *C. acaulis* EO and the *C. acaulis*-based NE were highly toxic to *L. botrana* larvae, with LC_{50} values of 7.299 and 9.044 µL/mL for *C. acaulis* EO and NE, respectively. The *C. acaulis*-based NE represents a promising option to develop highly stable botanical insecticides for pest management. To date, this study represents the first evidence about the insecticidal toxicity of EOs and EO-based NEs against this major grapevine pest.

Keywords: European grapevine moth; green pesticide; insect pest; Integrated Pest Management; Larvicide; nano-insecticide; Tortricidae

1. Introduction

The European grapevine moth (EGVM), *Lobesia botrana* (Denis & Schiffermüller, 1775) (Lepidoptera: Tortricidae), is a widespread and economically important pest of the grapevine worldwide. EGVM larvae feed on grape bunches (*Vitis vinifera* L.), reducing yield and increasing susceptibility to fungal and bacterial infections (i.e., botrytis and sour rot) [1].

Eco-friendly tools, including mating disruption and biopesticides (BPs) (mainly *Bacillus thuringiensis*), have been available against *L. botrana* for decades [2–5]. However, its control often requires the use of chemicals [6–9]. Finding valid and sustainable alternatives to insecticides is a key challenge for modern agriculture; side effects of insecticide use include environmental pollution, toxicity to non-target insects, and residues on food [10–13]. In this scenario, researchers are looking for new sustainable tools and products. Recently, they have focused on essential oils (EOs) as a new class of BPs to be employed in eco-friendly practices [14].

EOs are mixtures of plant metabolites, mainly monoterpenoids, sesquiterpenoids, and phenylpropanoids [14]; their insecticidal, acaricidal and nematocidal properties make them excellent alternatives to synthetic insecticides [14–16]. EOs are often characterized by two or three main compounds at high concentrations (20–85%) and other molecules at trace levels. A mechanism of action of EOs involves the inhibition of P450 cytochromes (i.e., these cytochromes are responsible for phase I metabolism of xenobiotics); other modes of actions include the neurotoxic activity-modulating octopaminergic system, gamma-aminobutyric acid (GABA) receptors and inhibiting acetylcholinesterase (AChE) [14].

EOs repellence [17,18], larvicidal [19–21], and insecticidal activities are proven on different arthropod pests of economic importance [22–25]. Among them, the EOs' efficacy has also been investigated on some Lepidoptera. Good examples are represented by *Cydia pomonella* (Linneaus) (Lepidoptera: Tortricidae) [26], *Thaumetopoea pityocampa* (Denis & Schiffermüller) (Lepidoptera: Notodontidae) [27], *Cadra cautella* (Walker) (Lepidoptera: Pyralidae) [28] as well as *Spodoptera littoralis* (Boisd.) [29–31] and *Spodoptera litura* (Fabr.) (Lepidoptera: Noctuidae) [32–34]. However, current knowledge about EOs toxicity on *L. botrana* larvae is strictly limited [35].

Even though EOs represent promising BP ingredients, their use in Integrated Pest Management (IPM) programs is still scarce because their physico-chemical properties (i.e., poor water solubility, scarce stability, high volatility, thermal decomposition, and oxidative degradation) make them difficult to handle in field conditions. A solution to these difficulties is to coat or entrap EOs into a matrix. The encapsulation process enhances physico-chemical stability, prevents degradation of active agents, and improves the bioavailability of EOs [36,37]. Nanotechnology represents a suitable strategy to carry the EOs' active principles, overcoming their physiochemical limitations; the small size of nano-systems increases active ingredients spreading, deposition, permeation, and provides controlled release on the target site. Among nano-delivery systems, nanoemulsions (NEs) represent an efficient, low-priced, and safe way to carry EOs [38].

As defined by Nikam et al. [39], NEs are kinetically stable "biphasic dispersions of two immiscible liquids: either water-in-oil (W/O) or oil-in-water (O/W) droplets stabilized by an amphiphilic surfactant"; in this way, protection from the surrounding environment, suitable spreading, and penetration of the bioactive molecules are guaranteed by the matrix and low surface and interfacial tension [40]. Toxicity of EO-based NEs was tested on several insects of agricultural and medical interest such as aphids [41–43], mosquitoes [44–46], stored-product beetles [47,48], and some Lepidoptera [49–51]. Furthermore, it was also highlighted that the bioactivity of EO-based NEs was often higher compared to the EOs themselves [52–54].

The insecticidal activity of EO-based NEs has been never evaluated against *L. botrana*. Herein, we decided to deepen our knowledge about EO and EO-based NE effectiveness against this harmful insect pest. For this purpose, we selected the EO obtained from the root of *Carlina acaulis* L. (Asteraceae), which has revealed to be promising as an active ingredient of botanical insecticides, highly effective against vectors and stored product insects [55,56].

Carlina acaulis, also called "piccolo cardo", is a perennial herb growing on the mountainous soils of central Europe, up to 2000 m of altitude [57]. Being described in several official pharmacopoeias [58–61], this plant has been largely used in the European tradition as a remedy against several diseases [62–64]. Nowadays, its traditional use is still recognised in many European countries as a tonic, diuretic, anti-oedematous, anticancer, and antibiotic agent, and for the treatment of gastritis and cold [65–68]. Along with its various curative applications, *C. acaulis* is also described in the Italian list of botanicals to be used in food supplements [69] and in the BELFRIT (Belgium France Italy) list [70]. The EO obtained from the roots of this plant revealed as a major constituent (>90%) the polyacetylene 2–(3–phenylprop–1–yn–1–yl)–furan, also known as carlina oxide. The biological activities shown by this EO are noteworthy, but its innovative insecticidal potential is attracting the interest of the agrochemical industry.

In this scenario, reminding the importance of botanical EOs for the development of new sustainable pesticides, considering the promising insecticidal activities showed by the *C. acaulis* EO [56,71], and the limitations linked with its lipophilicity and volatility as well, herein a highly stable *C. acaulis*-based NE was developed. Furthermore, the *C. acaulis* EO and *C. acaulis*-based NE were evaluated for their toxicity against 1st instar larvae of *L. botrana*, a major grape pest worldwide.

2. Materials and Methods

2.1. Carlina acaulis Oil Extraction and Chemical Characterization

One kg of dry roots of *C. acaulis* obtained from A. Minardi and Figli S.r.l. (48012 Bagnacavallo RA, Italy), was firstly crushed using a shredder (Albrigi, mod. E0585, Stallavena, Verona, Italy), for then being put into a 10 L round flask with 6 L of distilled water. The roots were then subjected to hydrodistillation using a Clevenger-type apparatus for 8 h and using a heating system consisting of a Falc MA mantle (Falc Instruments, Treviglio, Italy). The EO, which showed a pale orangish colour, was obtained in a 0.4% yield (*w/w*). After the hydrodistillation process, the EO was decanted and separated from the aqueous layer, then dehydrated with anhydrous Na_2SO_4. Finally, it was collected in a vial closed with a polytetrafluoroethylene (PTFE)/silicone cap and kept at −20 °C until chemical analysis and subsequent biological assays. For the chemical characterization of the *C. acaulis* EO, the analysis was conducted using an Agilent 6890N gas chromatograph furnished of a single quadrupole 5973N mass spectrometer and an auto-sampler 7863 (Agilent, Wilmingotn, DE). The column used for the separation was an HP-5 MS capillary column (30 m length, 0.25 mm i.d., 0.1 μm film thickness; 5% phenylmethylpolysiloxane), supplied by Agilent (Folsom, CA, USA). The column was allowed to reach initially a temperature of 60 °C for 5 min, then it was raised up to 200 °C at 4 °C/min and finally to 280 °C at 11 °C/min for 15 min. The temperature of the injector and detector was set at 280 °C. The mobile phase used was constituted of 99.9% of He, with a flow of 1 mL/min. Before injection, the EO was diluted 1:100 in *n*-hexane, and then 1 μL was injected in split mode (1:50). The peak acquisition was achieved with electron impact (EI, 70 eV) mode in the range 29–400 *m/z*. The chromatograms obtained were analysed using the MSD ChemStation software (Agilent, Version G1701DA D.01.00) and the NIST Mass Spectral Search Program for the NIST/EPA/NIH EI and NIST Tandem Mass Spectral Library v. 2.3. The retention index (RI) was calculated using a mix of *n*–alkanes (C_7–C_{30}, Sigma-Aldrich, Milan, Italy), using the Vanden Dool and Kratz formula [72].

2.2. Preparation and Characterization of Carlina acaulis Essential Oil (EO) Nanoemulsion

Carlina acaulis EO-based NE was obtained through a high-energy method by using a high-pressure homogenizer. It was prepared according to the procedure reported by Rosi Cappellani et al. [73]. Briefly, 6% (*w/w*) of *C. acaulis* EO was added dropwise to a 4% (*w/w*) of surfactant (Polysorbate 80, Sigma-Aldrich) aqueous solution under high-speed stirring (Ultraturrax T25 basic, IKA® Werke GmbH and Co.KG, Staufen, Germany) for 5 min at 9500 rpm. The obtained emulsion was then subjected to homogenization by means of a French Pressure Cell Press (American Instrument Company, AMINCO, Silver Spring, MD, USA) for four cycles at the pressure of 130 MPa.

Visual characterization of NE was performed by a polarizing optical microscope (MT9000, Meiji Techno Co. Ltd., Saitama, Japan) equipped with a 3-megapixel complementary metal oxide semiconductor (CMOS) sensor camera (Invenio 3S, DeltaPix, Smorum, Denmark).

Particle size measurements were carried out through dynamic light scattering (DLS) analyses by using a Zetasizer nanoS (Malvern Instrument, Malvern, UK) equipped with a backscattered light detector working at 173°. One mL of the sample was inserted into a disposable cuvette and analysed at 25 °C, following a temperature equilibration time (180 s).

2.3. Nanoemulsion Stability Studies

2.3.1. Long-Term Stability

The sample was stored at room temperature and 12:12 (L:D) h for up to six months. The physico-chemical stability of the samples was evaluated by repeating DLS analysis at different time points: 0 day (t0), 1 month (t1), 3 months (t3), and 6 months (t6).

2.3.2. Accelerated Stability Test

The thermodynamic stability of *C. acaulis* EO NE was evaluated through a three phases (centrifugation, heating/cooling cycles, and freeze/thaw cycles) test, according to the protocol reported by Alkilani et al. [74] with some modifications.

1. Centrifugation: the sample was centrifuged at 9000 G for 30 min. If it did not show any phase separation, the heating-cooling cycle was performed.
2. Heating-cooling cycle: the sample underwent three cycles from refrigerator temperature (4 °C) to 40 °C, with a storage period at each temperature of 48 h. If stable at these temperatures, the freeze-thaw cycle was performed.
3. Freeze-thaw cycle: three freeze-thaw cycles between −21 °C and +25 °C were performed, with a storage time at each temperature of 48 h.

At the end of each phase, the sample was evaluated through visual inspection and DLS analysis.

2.4. Lobesia botrana Mass-Rearing

Lobesia botrana young instars tested in our bioassays were from a laboratory mass-rearing kept at the Entomology lab, University of Pisa. Adults were reared inside a plastic bottle and fed with a liquid diet. Eggs were collected every 2 days and placed into a plastic tray, previously drilled to allow airflow; each tray contained a piece of artificial food medium. Semi-synthetic larval diet is based on Gabel et al. [75] recipe (for 1 kg: deionized water 750 mL, agar-agar 15 g, sucrose 30 g, alfalfa flour 25 g, brewer's yeast 18 g, salts of Wessen 12.5 g, cholesterol 1.25 g, wheat germ 90 g, casein 40 g, sorbic acid 2 g, ascorbic acid 10 g, vitamins wanderzahnt 7.5 g, tetracycline 1.25 g, propionic acid 2.5 g, linoleic acid 1 mL, sunflower oil 2 mL); emerged adults were transferred into a new polyvinyl chloride (PVC) bottle. The rearing was maintained at a temperature of 25 ± 1 °C, R.H. $70 \pm 10\%$ and 16:8 (L:D) photoperiod.

2.5. Insecticidal Activity on Lobesia botrana

The insecticidal activity of EO and NE of *C. acaulis* on *L. botrana* was tested adapting the method by Bosch et al. [76] originally developed for insecticide toxicity assessment on *C. pomonella*. A 32 µL-drop of NE or EO formulation was deposited on the surface of a piece of semi-synthetic diet ($4 \times 4 \times 1$ cm) using a micropipette. The solution was evenly distributed using a humidified brush and allowed to dry for 2 h. Sixteen 1st instar larvae (L1) of *L. botrana* were deposited on each piece of diet and individualized within a gelatine capsule (00, Fagron, Quarto Inferiore, Bologna, Italy). Each piece of the diet with the larvae was placed in a closed plastic box to avoid desiccation.

Larval mortality was observed 96 h later, gelatine capsules were removed, and the diet was observed under a binocular microscope for larvae inside the diet. A larva was considered dead if it did not respond to a gentle touch with a small brush. Missing larvae were considered escaped and subtracted from the number of treated larvae. Seven concentrations of *C. acaulis* EO (1, 2.5, 6, 7.5, 8, 10, 30 µL/mL) and six concentrations of *C. acaulis* NE (5, 7.5, 8, 10, 30, 60 µL/mL) were tested, water was used as solvent to prepare the dilutions.

To validate the method described above, we also tested positive and negative controls. The positive control was a commercial insecticide, Spinosad (Laser®, Dow) tested at the tab dose (15 mL/hL); the negative control was 0.17% Polysorbate 80 + 99.83% of H_2O for NE and H_2O + dimethyl sulfoxide (DMSO) at the same concentration of the EO. At least three replicas for each concentration of EO, NE, positive and negative control were performed. For each tested product concentration, four duplicate trials were carried out; replicates were conducted over different days to account for any daily variability. Each concentration was always replicated with a new concentration series prepared for each replicate. All experiments were performed at laboratory conditions of 22 ± 1 °C, R.H. 45 ± 5%, and photoperiod 16:8 (L:D).

2.6. Statistical Analysis

Lobesia botrana mortality (%) was arcsine$\sqrt{}$ transformed before performing an analysis of variance (ANOVA, two factors as fixed effects) followed by Tukey's honestly significant difference (HSD) test ($p < 0.05$). The experimental mortality was corrected with Abbott's formula, if control mortality ranged from 1 to 20%; if control mortality was > 20% experiments were discarded and repeated [77]. LC_{10}, LC_{30}, LC_{50}, and LC_{90} with associated 95% confidence interval (CI) and chi-squares, were estimated using probit analysis [78]. JMP9 (SAS) software was used for all analyses, and $p = 0.05$ was selected as a threshold to assess significant differences.

3. Results and Discussion

3.1. Essential Oil Chemical Composition

Through gas chromatography–mass spectrometry (GC–MS) analysis, the EO extracted from the roots of *C. acaulis* was characterised and the data obtained were in accordance with the work of Benelli et al. [56]. Seven compounds were identified, among which carlina oxide was the predominant EO component, comprising 94.6% of the relative content. Other compounds were identified, such as the aromatic benzaldehyde (3.1%) and the sesquiterpene *ar*-curcumene (0.4%) (Figure 1). Acetophenone, benzyl methyl ketone, camphor, and carvone were detected at trace levels.

3.2. Preparation and Characterization of the Essential Oil Nanoemulsion

NEs are colloidal systems offering a great advantage to encapsulate a higher amount of oil phase respective to similar nanosystems, i.e., microemulsions [79]. In fact, such a system has allowed to vehiculate 6% (*w/w*) of EO, respective to at least 1.5% (*w/w*) encapsulated into microemulsions, as reported in previous studies [80,81]. Moreover, NEs require a meager amount of surfactant (4% *w/w*), with a surfactant-to-oil ratio (SOR) of around 0.6, respective to that of microemulsions, that is generally higher than 2 (SOR > 2) [82].

However, NEs are energetically disadvantaged nanosystems because they have a higher free energy level respective to that of the two separated phases (water + oil). Thus, to produce a colloidal system, an external energetic input is required to overcome the activation energy barrier separating the two phases. In this respect, one of the most commonly used methods is the homogenization process. It is a high-energy method that consists of a 2-step procedure [83]. The first step gives rise to an emulsion, characterized by oil droplets mainly in the micrometric range, through the high-speed stirring process of the oil and water phases [82]. The second step, the high-pressure homogenization, provides the breakage of oil droplets into small ones by forcing the material to flow through small nozzles or valves by exerting very high pressures with a piston pump. During the flow, the emulsion is exposed to shear stress able to give rise to nanometric oily droplets [84].

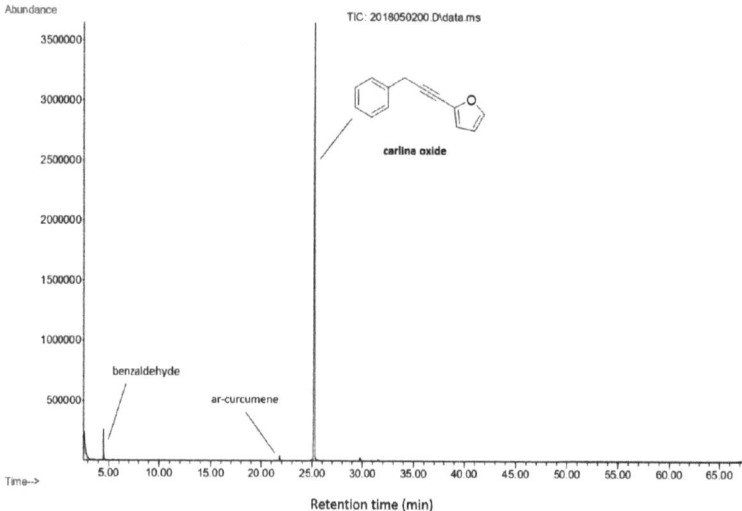

Figure 1. Gas chromatography–mass spectrometry (GC–MS) chromatogram of the essential oil obtained from the roots of *Carlina acaulis*. The separation of peaks was achieved using a HP-5MS (5% phenylmethylpolysiloxane, 30 m length × 0.25 mm internal diameter, 0.1 µm film thickness).

For the achievement of *C. acaulis* EO-based NE, the sample was subjected to a pressure of 130 MPa four times. The sample showed a monomodal size distribution with a size in the nanometric range. In particular, the droplets' population had a mean diameter centred around 140 nm (Figure 2, black line). DLS analysis recorded Z-average and PDI (polydispersity index) values of 98.85 and 0.33, respectively. The Z-average value or Z-average mean used in DLS is a parameter, also known as the cumulants mean, that can be defined as the "harmonic intensity averaged particle diameter". Assuming that the particle population is a simple Gaussian distribution, the Z-average is the mean, and the PDI is related to the width of this simple distribution. Thus, the smaller the PDI (≤ 0.3), the more monodispersed the system will be [85].

The *C. acaulis* EO NE showed optimal stability at room temperature, evaluated for a storage period of six months. As reported in Figure 2, the size of the oil droplets remained almost unchanged, with a slight shift of mean hydrodynamic diameter from 143.9 nm at t0 to 170.2 nm after 6 months. These results proved the thermodynamic stability of the system. It was also confirmed by the accelerated stability test, generally used to predict the thermodynamic stability of the system for long-term periods. The accelerated stability was evaluated via centrifugation, heating–cooling cycles, and finally, freeze-thaw cycles stress tests. The NE showed a good physical stability at the centrifugal forces (Figure 3B) and remained almost unaltered to the heat–cool cycles. No signs of creaming, phase separation or cracking were detected (Figure 3C). These images were also corroborated by DLS analysis results (Table 1), that revealed the conservation of the internal phase structure, being the Z-average and PDI values almost unchanged with respect to those of the NE at t0. A slight creaming effect was observed when the NE was frozen at the temperature of −21 °C. However, its homogeneity was recovered upon the thawing phase (Figure 3D). A similar result was reported by Ammar et al. [86], who attributed this transient instability to the low temperature leading to the coagulation of the internal phase. This perturbation of the systems was revealed by the increased value of the Z-average after the freeze-thaw cycles, as reported in Table 1. However, the size of the oil phase was kept below 200 nm, which is the upper limit generally established by authors for NEs [87].

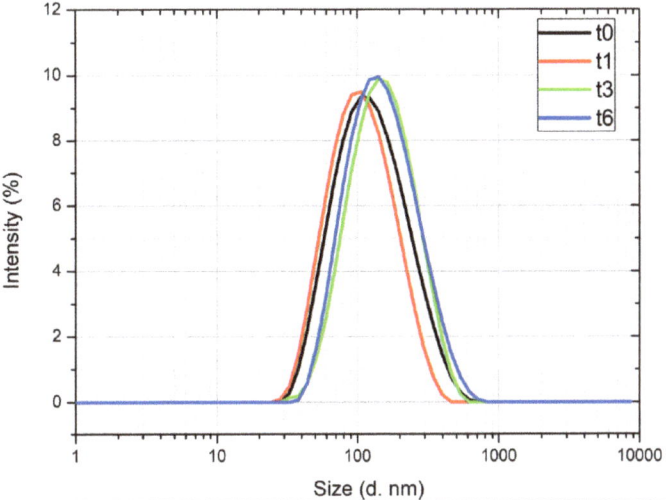

Figure 2. Dynamic light scattering (DLS) traces of *Carlina acaulis* essential oil-based nanoemulsion, at different time points: 0 day (t0), 1 month (t1), 3 months (t3), 6 months (t6).

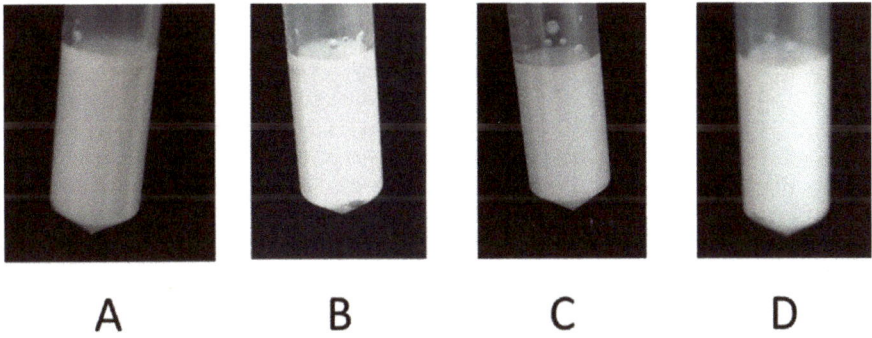

Figure 3. *Carlina acaulis* essential oil nanoemulsion (EO NE) at t0 (**A**), after the centrifugation (**B**), after the heating–cooling cycles (**C**) and after the freeze-thaw cycles (**D**).

Table 1. Thermodynamic stability evaluation, in terms of Z-average, polydispersity index (PDI), creaming, and phase separation, of the *Carlina acaulis* essential oil (EO) nanoemulsion through the accelerated stability test.

	Z-Average *	SD	PDI *	SD	Creaming	Phase Separation
t0	98.85	1.41	0.33	0.04	-	-
Post CENTRIFUGATION	95.54	1.32	0.31	0.031	NO	NO
Post HEATING-COOLING	90.68	1.32	0.33	0.02	NO	NO
Post FREEZE-THAW	153.93	1.58	0.28	0.005	NO **	NO

* The value is the mean of three measurements. ** The creaming phenomenon was observed only after the freezing of the sample. However, at the end of the cycles, after the thawing process, the sample did not more show creaming.

Therefore, given the results achieved by the stability study, this *C. acaulis* EO-based NE can be considered a physico-chemically stable nanosystem.

3.3. Insecticidal Activity on Lobesia botrana

Larval mortality in exposed *L. botrana* individuals was directly proportional to *C. acaulis* EO and *C. acaulis*-based NE concentrations ($F_{6,23} = 40.47$, $p < 0.0001$; $F_{5,23} = 27.22$, $p < 0.0001$, respectively); significant larvicidal activity was observed starting from 2.5 µL/mL of EO and 8.0 µL/mL of NE. Comparable concentrations of *C. acaulis* EO showed higher larvicidal activity over the *C. acaulis* EO NE. As reported in Table 2, 50% of larval mortality was achieved testing a concentration equal to 7.29 ± 0.25 µL/mL of *C. acaulis* EO and 9.04 ± 0.39 µL/mL of *C. acaulis* NE. Besides, the LC_{90} of *C. acaulis* EO was lower than that of *C. acaulis*-based NE (10.92 ± 1.40 µL/mL and 17.70 ± 4.48 µL/mL, respectively); 100% larval mortality was achieved with the positive control represented by a semi-synthetic diet treated with the positive control spinosad (Laser®) at the label dose (i.e., 150 ppm).

Table 2. Larvicidal activity of *Carlina acaulis* essential oil (EO) and its 6% nanoemulsion (NE) against 1st instar larvae of *Lobesia botrana*.

Tested Product	LC_{10}[1] ± SE[2] (CI_{95})[3] (µL/mL)	LC_{30} ± SE (CI_{95}) (µL/mL)	LC_{50} ± SE (CI_{95}) (µL/mL)	LC_{90} ± SE (CI_{95}) (µL/mL)	χ^2	*p*-Value
C. acaulis EO	4.87 ± 0.49 (3.9–5.4)	6.19 ± 0.31 (5.6–6.5)	7.29 ± 0.25 (6.9–7.6)	10.92 ± 1.40 (9.7–13.6)	1.158	0.563 n.s.[4]
C. acaulis EO in NE	6.24 ± 0.58 (5.1–6.8)	7.77 ± 0.33 (7.2–8.1)	9.04 ± 0.39 (8.6–9.7)	17.70 ± 4.48 (15.4–27.5)	1.257	0.262 n.s.

[1] LC = lethal concentration killing 10%(LC_{10}), 30% (LC_{30}), 50%(LC_{50}) or 90% (LC_{90}) of the exposed population; [2] SE = standard error; [3] CI_{95} = 95% confidence interval; [4] n.s. = not significant ($p > 0.05$). Positive control spinosad (Laser®) tested at tab dose (150 ppm) achieved 100% mortality.

It is difficult to compare our results with the findings by other authors as, to the best of our knowledge, research on the insecticidal efficacy of plant EOs against *L. botrana* is extremely limited. Only one study was retrieved, where Avgin et al. [35] tested 5 essential oils from seeds or aerial parts of aromatic plants such as *Thymus vulgaris* L., *Mentha x piperita* L., *Foeniculum vulgare* Mill., *Rosmarinus officinalis* L. and *Carum carvi* L. on field-collected grapes. The authors found that the EO from *C. carvi* was the most effective, since at a concentration of 25 µL on 20 g of grapes it achieved >96% mortality on *L. botrana* larvae. Most research about the EO efficacy on *L. botrana* was undertaken to explore any changes in adults' behaviour in response to EO aroma [88], aimed at using EOs to improve pest control strategies [89]. As far as we know, our study is the first that assesses EO efficacy on the mortality of freshly hatched *L. botrana* larvae as the usual target of insecticide application. Also, the study of EO-based NE efficacy on the larvae of phytophagous lepidopteran species is only beginning, and few papers on NE efficacy on moth pests exist so far [49–51], although EOs have been known to provide very good insecticidal effects on pests including phytophagous moth larvae [26,27]. Moreover, as indicated by previous studies, EO-based NEs actually show very promising effects, often significantly higher if compared to EOs [49,52,53].

Carlina acaulis EO was obtained from roots of carline thistle, and its main component is carlina oxide (~94%), one of the oldest known polyacetylenes. A recent study conducted by Benelli et al. [56] proved carlina oxide as a mild acetylcholinesterase (AChE) inhibitor. It has also been documented that polyacetylenes cause phototoxicity in insects [90], and are able to modulate $GABA_A$ receptors [91]. Recently, the effectiveness of *C. acaulis* EO has been demonstrated on other insect species, showing acute and sub-lethal toxicity on highly important pests and vectors, such as the southern house mosquito, *Culex quinquefasciatus* (Say) (Diptera: Culicidae) (LC_{50} = 1.31 µg mL^{-1}) [56] and the common housefly, *Musca domestica* (L.) (Diptera: Muscidae) (LC_{50} = 2.74 (♂) and 5.96 (♀) µg fly^{-1}) [71]. Moreover, simulating a small-scale maize conservation environment, the *C. acaulis* EO led to relevant insecticidal activity against *Prostephanus truncatus* (Horn) (Coleoptera: Bostrychidae), with 500 ppm killing >97% of adult beetles within three days [55]. Either the effectiveness, as well as the availability and low costs of the *C. acaulis* EO, encourage further experimentation on EGVM for green pesticide development.

The comparison of the LC values obtained by testing *C. acaulis* EO and the corresponding NE, showed a comparable larvicidal activity. From the values reported in Table 2, it is possible to observe a higher insecticidal activity of the pure EO (LC_{90} = 10.922 ± 1.40 µL/mL) over the NE (LC_{90} = 17.706 ± 4.48 µL/mL). On the other hand, the NE contains 6% of EO, a value 16 times lower respect to pure EO used as reference. This shows that the EO encapsulated in the NE is more active than the pure *C. acaulis* EO, if considered at the same concentration. The increase in the larvicidal activity of pure EO encapsulated into the NE could be attributed to a better interaction between the active substance and the target site. First, the NE, providing a greater dispersion of the lipophilic substance (EO) in the aqueous phase, allows the diffusion of the EO in the *L. botrana* growth environment. Furthermore, the NE is able to increase the concentration of the EO at the interface, leading to a better and direct interaction with the biological components of the target. Moreover, the small size and large surface area of the NE-encapsulated EO droplets allow an increased absorption and cellular penetration into the target site. Therefore, the encapsulated EO can exert its larvicidal activity even at lower concentrations than pure EO. Finally, the NE appears promising in controlling the growth of *L. botrana*, not only for the larvicidal potential but also for the improvement of the physico-chemical properties and stability of the EO [38].

The efficacy of EOs including EO-based NEs may not be necessarily related only to acute or chronic toxicity, but, as already shown, even sub-lethal EO doses or concentrations may reduce the vitality, fertility, and longevity of insects [92,93] including harmful moths [26–28]. This phenomenon was also confirmed for the EO from *C. acaulis*, although for other insect species [56,71] and, therefore, any potential effect of sub-lethal concentrations should be studied for *L. botrana* as well. Similarly, the possibility of enhancing the insecticidal activity of the EO from *C. acaulis* using a suitable synergistic mixture with other EOs or their major constituents should be considered in further studies.

This study opens a new perspective on *L. botrana* management using botanical pesticides. It highlights the potential of Asteraceae EOs as valid alternatives to chemical insecticides, because of their low human toxicity, rapid degradation, low environmental impact, and reduced likelihood to trigger insecticide resistance [14,94,95]. The lack of physico-chemical stability makes EOs difficult to handle in open field conditions. However, the adoption of nano-delivery systems (e.g., NEs) increases EOs stability and solubility, improving their delivery, and establishing a sustained release of the active ingredients [38]. The adoption of nanotechnology in IPM showed it to be useful to overcome EOs' drawbacks and to amend their efficacy as biopesticides.

Further studies should be conducted on the larvicidal and adulticidal activity of EOs and EO-based NEs on *L. botrana* to find a valid substance to test in the open field. Moreover, as highlighted by Pavoni et al. [79], it is crucial to consider that a lot of EO-based NEs contain several, non eco-friendly ingredients (i.e., polysorbates). Thus, further research is needed to evaluate the effects of nano-encapsulation on EO toxicological profiles.

As mentioned above, the use of EOs to eliminate insects is an alternative pest control method that minimises any harmful effects on the environment. Since EOs are chemicals commonly found in nature, being contained in almost all vascular plants, and have been shown to be very friendly to non-target organisms, botanical insecticides based on EOs can be considered relatively safe for the environment [14,38,94]. Moreover, as EOs are highly volatile, only minimal problems with their residues are expected when used in soil and aquatic ecosystems [94]. We are aware that further studies on the effects of *C. acaulis* EO on non-target organisms will be needed to confirm environmental safety for this EO. Although solvents are usually added to EO-based formulations [79], NEs used in this study contain no solvents and are based on a surfactant with no effects in terms of eco-toxicity given its high level of biodegradability.

4. Conclusions

The present study highlighted the promising potential of the *C. acaulis* root EO as an effective ingredient for botanical insecticide development. This EO showed high insecticidal efficacy against 1st instar larvae of *L. botrana*, a major pest affecting grape cultivation, causing yearly significant economic damages. Moreover, this research supported the real-world applications of the *C. acaulis* EO through its encapsulation into a nanoformulation. The EO-based NE guarantees the conservation of the insecticidal activity while ensuring dispersibility in the environment as well as its stability along time. Although the results encourage the use of *C. acaulis* EO in the agricultural field, especially in organic farming, further investigations are needed to evaluate its eco-toxicological profile. Similarly, further studies are needed to reveal the effects of lethal and sub-lethal concentrations on fertility, longevity, and behaviour of *L. botrana*.

Author Contributions: Conceptualization, G.B. (Giovanni Benelli), L.P., G.B. (Giulia Bonacucina), F.M., and A.L.; methodology, G.B. (Giovanni Benelli), L.P., V.Z., R.R., E.S., S.G., R.P. (Roman Pavela), G.B. (Giulia Bonacucina) and F.M.; software, G.B. (Giovanni Benelli) and R.P. (Roman Pavela); validation, G.B. (Giovanni Benelli), L.P., R.P. (Roman Pavela), R.P. (Riccardo Petrelli) L.C., F.M., G.B. (Giulia Bonacucina) and A.L.; formal analysis, G.B. (Giovanni Benelli), L.P., V.Z., R.R., F.C., G.C., E.S., S.G., R.P. (Roman Pavela), R.P. (Riccardo Petrelli), L.C., F.M., G.B. (Giulia Bonacucina) and A.L.; investigation, G.B. (Giovanni Benelli), L.P., V.Z., R.R., F.C., G.C., E.S., S.G., F.M., and A.L.; resources, G.B. (Giovanni Benelli), G.B. (Giulia Bonacucina), R.P. (Riccardo Petrelli), L.C., and F.M.; data curation, G.B., L.P., R.P. (Roman Pavela), F.M., G.B. (Giulia Bonacucina), V.Z.; writing—original draft preparation, G.B. (Giovanni Benelli), L.P., V.Z., G.B. (Giulia Bonacucina), F.M. and A.L.; writing—review and editing, G.B. (Giovanni Benelli), L.P., V.Z., R.R., F.C., G.C., E.S., S.G., R.P. (Roman Pavela), R.P. (Riccardo Petrelli), L.C., F.M., G.B. (Giulia Bonacucina) and A.L.; visualization, G.B. (Giovanni Benelli), L.P., V.Z., R.R., F.C., G.C., E.S., S.G., R.P. (Roman Pavela), R.P. (Riccardo Petrelli), L.C., F.M., G.B. (Giulia Bonacucina) and A.L.; supervision, G.B. (Giovanni Benelli), G.B. (Giulia Bonacucina), F.M., R.P. (Riccardo Petrelli), R.P. (Roman Pavela), G.B. (Giulia Bonacucina) and A.L.; funding acquisition, G.B. (Giovanni Benelli), R.P. (Roman Pavela), and R.P. (Riccardo Petrelli) All authors have read and agreed to the published version of the manuscript.

Funding: Riccardo Petrelli would like to thank the Italian Ministry of Health for the PRIN grant (PRIN 2017,2017CBNCYT_005) for financial support. Roman Pavela would like to thank the Ministry of Agriculture of the Czech Republic for its financial support concerning botanical pesticide and basic substances research (Project MZE-RO0418).

Acknowledgments: We are grateful to Patrizia Mazzarisi and Paolo Giannotti (University of Pisa, Italy) for their technical assistance in *L. botrana* rearing.

Conflicts of Interest: The authors declare no conflict of interest.

References

1. Ioriatti, C.; Anfora, G.; Tasin, M.; De Cristofaro, A.; Witzgall, P.; Lucchi, A. Chemical Ecology and Management of *Lobesia botrana* (Lepidoptera: Tortricidae). *J. Econ. Entomol.* **2011**, *104*, 1125–1137. [CrossRef]
2. Lucchi, A.; Benelli, G. Towards pesticide-free farming? Sharing needs and knowledge promotes Integrated Pest Management. *Environ. Sci. Pollut. Res.* **2018**, *25*, 13439–13445. [CrossRef]
3. Benelli, G.; Lucchi, A.; Thomson, D.; Ioriatti, C. Sex Pheromone Aerosol Devices for Mating Disruption: Challenges for a Brighter Future. *Insects* **2019**, *10*, 308. [CrossRef]
4. Lucchi, A.; Sambado, P.; Juan Royo, A.B.; Bagnoli, B.; Conte, G.; Benelli, G. Disrupting mating of *Lobesia botrana* using sex pheromone aerosol devices. *Environ. Sci. Pollut. Res.* **2018**, *25*, 22196–22204. [CrossRef]
5. Ifoulis, A.A.; Savopoulou-Soultani, M. Biological control of *Lobesia botrana* (Lepidoptera: Tortricidae) larvae by using different formulations of *Bacillus thuringiensis* in 11 vine cultivars under field conditions. *J. Econ. Entomol.* **2004**, *97*, 340–343. [CrossRef]
6. Civolani, S.; Boselli, M.; Butturini, A.; Chicca, M.; Fano, E.A.; Cassanelli, S. Assessment of insecticide resistance of *Lobesia botrana* (Lepidoptera: Tortricidae) in Emilia-Romagna region. *J. Econ. Entomol.* **2014**, *107*, 1245–1249. [CrossRef]
7. Vassiliou, V.A. Effectiveness of insecticides in controlling the first and second generations of the *Lobesia botrana* (Lepidoptera: Tortricidae) in table grapes. *J. Econ. Entomol.* **2011**, *104*, 580–585. [CrossRef]
8. Pavan, F.; Cargnus, E.; Bigot, G.; Zandigiacomo, P. Residual activity of insecticides applied against *Lobesia botrana* and its influence on resistance management strategies. *Bull. Insectol.* **2014**, *67*, 273–280.

9. Thiéry, D.; Louâpre, P.; Muneret, L.; Rusch, A.; Sentenac, G.; Vogelweith, F.; Iltis, C.; Moreau, J. Biological protection against grape berry moths. A review. *Agron. Sustain. Dev.* **2018**, *38*, 15. [CrossRef]
10. Desneux, N.; Decourtye, A.; Delpuech, J.-M. The Sublethal Effects of Pesticides on Beneficial Arthropods. *Annu. Rev. Entomol.* **2006**, *52*, 81–106. [CrossRef]
11. Guedes, R.N.C. Insecticide resistance, control failure likelihood and the First Law of Geography. *Pest Manag. Sci.* **2017**, *73*, 479–484. [CrossRef] [PubMed]
12. Navarro Roldán, M.; Gemeno, C. Sublethal Effects of Neonicotinoid Insecticide on Calling Behavior and Pheromone Production of Tortricid Moths. *J. Chem. Ecol.* **2017**, *43*, 881–890. [CrossRef] [PubMed]
13. Benelli, G. Plant-borne compounds and nanoparticles: Challenges for medicine, parasitology and entomology. *Environ. Sci. Pollut. Res.* **2018**, *25*, 10149–10150. [CrossRef] [PubMed]
14. Pavela, R.; Benelli, G. Essential Oils as Ecofriendly Biopesticides? Challenges and Constraints. *Trends Plant. Sci.* **2016**, *21*, 1000–1007. [CrossRef] [PubMed]
15. Bakkali, F.; Averbeck, S.; Averbeck, D.; Idaomar, M. Biological effects of essential oils—A review. *Food Chem. Toxicol.* **2008**, *46*, 446–475. [CrossRef] [PubMed]
16. Li, Y.; Fabiano-Tixier, A.-S.; Chemat, F. Essential Oils: From Conventional to Green Extraction. In *Essential Oils as Reagents in Green Chemistry*; Li, Y., Fabiano-Tixier, A.-S., Chemat, F., Eds.; SpringerBriefs in Molecular Science; Springer International Publishing: Cham, Switzerland, 2014; pp. 9–20, ISBN 978-3-319-08449-7.
17. Nerio, L.S.; Olivero-Verbel, J.; Stashenko, E. Repellent activity of essential oils: A review. *Bioresour. Technol.* **2010**, *101*, 372–378. [CrossRef]
18. de Souza, M.A.; da Silva, L.; Macêdo, M.J.F.; Lacerda-Neto, L.J.; dos Santos, M.A.C.; Coutinho, H.D.M.; Cunha, F.A.B. Adulticide and repellent activity of essential oils against *Aedes aegypti* (Diptera: Culicidae)—A review. *S. Afr. J. Bot.* **2019**, *124*, 160–165. [CrossRef]
19. Kanat, M.; Alma, M.H. Insecticidal effects of essential oils from various plants against larvae of pine processionary moth (*Thaumetopoea pityocampa* Schiff) (Lepidoptera: Thaumetopoeidae). *Pest Manag. Sci.* **2004**, *60*, 173–177. [CrossRef]
20. Pavela, R.; Maggi, F.; Cianfaglione, K.; Bruno, M.; Benelli, G. Larvicidal Activity of Essential Oils of Five Apiaceae Taxa and Some of Their Main Constituents Against *Culex quinquefasciatus*. *Chem. Biodivers.* **2018**, *15*, e1700382. [CrossRef]
21. Chandrasekaran, T.; Thyagarajan, A.; Santhakumari, P.G.; Pillai, A.K.B.; Krishnan, U.M. Larvicidal activity of essential oil from *Vitex negundo* and *Vitex trifolia* on dengue vector mosquito *Aedes aegypti*. *Rev. Soc. Bras. Med. Trop.* **2019**, *52*. [CrossRef]
22. Ríos, N.; Stashenko, E.E.; Duque, J.E.; Ríos, N.; Stashenko, E.E.; Duque, J.E. Evaluation of the insecticidal activity of essential oils and their mixtures against *Aedes aegypti* (Diptera: Culicidae). *Rev. Bras. Entomol.* **2017**, *61*, 307–311. [CrossRef]
23. Pavela, R.; Žabka, M.; Bednář, J.; Tříska, J.; Vrchotová, N. New knowledge for yield, composition and insecticidal activity of essential oils obtained from the aerial parts or seeds of fennel (*Foeniculum vulgare* Mill.). *Ind. Crops Prod.* **2016**, *83*, 275–282. [CrossRef]
24. Filomeno, C.A.; Barbosa, L.C.A.; Teixeira, R.R.; Pinheiro, A.L.; de Sá Farias, E.; de Paula Silva, E.M.; Picanço, M.C. *Corymbia* spp. and *Eucalyptus* spp. essential oils have insecticidal activity against *Plutella xylostella*. *Ind. Crops Prod.* **2017**, *109*, 374–383. [CrossRef]
25. Benelli, G.; Pavela, R.; Rakotosaona, R.; Nzekoue, F.K.; Canale, A.; Nicoletti, M.; Maggi, F. Insecticidal and mosquito repellent efficacy of the essential oils from stem bark and wood of *Hazomalania voyronii*. *J. Ethnopharmacol.* **2020**, *248*, 112333. [CrossRef] [PubMed]
26. Landolt, P.J.; Hofstetter, R.W.; Biddick, L.L. Plant essential oils as arrestants and repellents for neonate larvae of the codling moth (Lepidoptera: Tortricidae). *Environ. Entomol.* **1999**, *28*, 954–960. [CrossRef]
27. Yigit, Ş.; Saruhan, İ.; Akça, İ. The effect of some commercial plant oils on the pine processionary moth *Thaumetopoea pityocampa* (Lepidoptera: Notodontidae). *J. For. Sci.* **2019**, *65*, 309–312. [CrossRef]
28. Gotyal, B.S.; Srivastava, C.; Walia, S. Fumigant Toxicity of Essential Oil from *Lantana camara* Against Almond Moth, *Cadra cautella* (Walker). *J. Essent. Oil Bear. Plants* **2016**, *19*, 1521–1526. [CrossRef]
29. Pavela, R.; Maggi, F.; Lupidi, G.; Cianfaglione, K.; Dauvergne, X.; Bruno, M.; Benelli, G. Efficacy of sea fennel (*Crithmum maritimum* L., Apiaceae) essential oils against *Culex quinquefasciatus* Say and *Spodoptera littoralis* (Boisd.). *Ind. Crops Prod.* **2017**, *109*, 603–610. [CrossRef]

30. Benelli, G.; Pavela, R.; Petrelli, R.; Cappellacci, L.; Santini, G.; Fiorini, D.; Sut, S.; Dall'Acqua, S.; Canale, A.; Maggi, F. The essential oil from industrial hemp (*Cannabis sativa* L.) by-products as an effective tool for insect pest management in organic crops. *Ind. Crops Prod.* **2018**, *122*, 308–315. [CrossRef]
31. Benelli, G.; Pavela, R.; Zorzetto, C.; Sánchez-Mateo, C.C.; Santini, G.; Canale, A.; Maggi, F. Insecticidal activity of the essential oil from *Schizogyne sericea* (Asteraceae) on four insect pests and two non-target species. *Entomol. Gen.* **2019**, 9–18. [CrossRef]
32. Vasantha-Srinivasan, P.; Senthil-Nathan, S.; Thanigaivel, A.; Edwin, E.-S.; Ponsankar, A.; Selin-Rani, S.; Pradeepa, V.; Sakthi-Bhagavathy, M.; Kalaivani, K.; Hunter, W.B.; et al. Developmental response of *Spodoptera litura* Fab. to treatments of crude volatile oil from *Piper betle* L. and evaluation of toxicity to earthworm, *Eudrilus eugeniae* Kinb. *Chemosphere* **2016**, *155*, 336–347. [CrossRef] [PubMed]
33. Selin-Rani, S.; Senthil-Nathan, S.; Thanigaivel, A.; Vasantha-Srinivasan, P.; Edwin, E.-S.; Ponsankar, A.; Lija-Escaline, J.; Kalaivani, K.; Abdel-Megeed, A.; Hunter, W.B.; et al. Toxicity and physiological effect of quercetin on generalist herbivore, *Spodoptera litura* Fab. and a non-target earthworm *Eisenia fetida* Savigny. *Chemosphere* **2016**, *165*, 257–267. [CrossRef] [PubMed]
34. Ponsankar, A.; Vasantha-Srinivasan, P.; Senthil-Nathan, S.; Thanigaivel, A.; Edwin, E.-S.; Selin-Rani, S.; Kalaivani, K.; Hunter, W.B.; Alessandro, R.T.; Abdel-Megeed, A.; et al. Target and non-target toxicity of botanical insecticide derived from *Couroupita guianensis* L. flower against generalist herbivore, *Spodoptera litura* Fab. and an earthworm, *Eisenia foetida* Savigny. *Ecotoxicol. Environ. Saf.* **2016**, *133*, 260–270. [CrossRef] [PubMed]
35. Avgın, S.S.; Karaman, Ş.; Bahadıroğlu, C. Laboratory Assays of Plant Extracts Against *Lobesia botrana* (Denis & Schiffermüller) (Lepidoptera: Tortricidae) Larvae. *J. Entomol. Sci.* **2008**, *43*, 423–425. [CrossRef]
36. Perlatti, B.; de Souza Bergo, P.L.; das Gracas Fernandes da Silva, M.F.; Batista Fernandes, J.; Rossi Forim, M. Polymeric Nanoparticle-Based Insecticides: A Controlled Release Purpose for Agrochemicals. In *Insecticides—Development of Safer and More Effective Technologies*; Trdan, S., Ed.; InTech: Rijeka, Croatia, 2013; pp. 521–548. [CrossRef]
37. Song, S.; Liu, X.; Jiang, J.; Qian, Y.; Zhang, N.; Wu, Q. Stability of triazophos in self-nanoemulsifying pesticide delivery system. *Colloids Surf. Physicochem. Eng. Asp.* **2009**, *350*, 57–62. [CrossRef]
38. Pavoni, L.; Pavela, R.; Cespi, M.; Bonacucina, G.; Maggi, F.; Zeni, V.; Canale, A.; Lucchi, A.; Bruschi, F.; Benelli, G. Green Micro- and Nanoemulsions for Managing Parasites, Vectors and Pests. *Nanomaterials* **2019**, *9*, 1285. [CrossRef]
39. Nikam, T.; Patil, M.; Patil, S.; Vadnere, G.; Lodhi, S. Nanoemulsion: A brief review on development and application in Parenteral Drug Delivery. *Adv. Pharm. J.* **2018**, *3*, 43–54. [CrossRef]
40. Turek, C.; Stintzing, F.C. Stability of Essential Oils: A Review. *Compr. Rev. Food Sci. Food Saf.* **2013**, *12*, 40–53. [CrossRef]
41. Heydari, M.; Amirjani, A.; Bagheri, M.; Sharifian, I.; Sabahi, Q. Eco-friendly pesticide based on peppermint oil nanoemulsion: Preparation, physicochemical properties, and its aphicidal activity against cotton aphid. *Environ. Sci. Pollut. Res.* **2020**, *27*, 6667–6679. [CrossRef]
42. Pascual-Villalobos, M.J.; Cantó-Tejero, M.; Vallejo, R.; Guirao, P.; Rodríguez-Rojo, S.; Cocero, M.J. Use of nanoemulsions of plant essential oils as aphid repellents. *Ind. Crops Prod.* **2017**, *110*, 45–57. [CrossRef]
43. Pascual-Villalobos, M.J.; Guirao, P.; Díaz-Baños, F.G.; Cantó-Tejero, M.; Villora, G. Oil in water nanoemulsion formulations of botanical active substances. In *Nano-Biopesticides Today and Future Perspectives*; Koul, O., Ed.; Academic Press: Cambridge, MA, USA, 2019; Chapter 9; pp. 223–247. [CrossRef]
44. Oliveira, A.E.M.F.M.; Duarte, J.L.; Cruz, R.A.S.; Souto, R.N.P.; Ferreira, R.M.A.; Peniche, T.; da Conceição, E.C.; de Oliveira, L.A.R.; Faustino, S.M.M.; Florentino, A.C.; et al. *Pterodon emarginatus* oleoresin-based nanoemulsion as a promising tool for *Culex quinquefasciatus* (Diptera: Culicidae) control. *J. Nanobiotechnol.* **2017**, *15*, 2. [CrossRef] [PubMed]
45. Duarte, J.L.; Amado, J.R.R.; Oliveira, A.E.M.F.M.; Cruz, R.A.S.; Ferreira, A.M.; Souto, R.N.P.; Falcão, D.Q.; Carvalho, J.C.T.; Fernandes, C.P. Evaluation of larvicidal activity of a nanoemulsion of *Rosmarinus officinalis* essential oil. *Rev. Bras. Farmacogn.* **2015**, *25*, 189–192. [CrossRef]
46. Sugumar, S.; Clarke, S.K.; Nirmala, M.J.; Tyagi, B.K.; Mukherjee, A.; Chandrasekaran, N. Nanoemulsion of eucalyptus oil and its larvicidal activity against *Culex quinquefasciatus*. *Bull. Entomol. Res.* **2014**, *104*, 393–402. [CrossRef] [PubMed]

47. Pant, M.; Dubey, S.; Patanjali, P.K.; Naik, S.N.; Sharma, S. Insecticidal activity of eucalyptus oil nanoemulsion with karanja and jatropha aqueous filtrates. *Int. Biodeterior. Biodegrad.* **2014**, *91*, 119–127. [CrossRef]
48. Choupanian, M.; Omar, D.; Basri, M.; Asib, N. Preparation and characterization of neem oil nanoemulsion formulations against *Sitophilus oryzae* and *Tribolium castaneum* adults. *J. Pestic. Sci.* **2017**, *42*, 158–165. [CrossRef]
49. Jesser, E.; Lorenzetti, A.S.; Yeguerman, C.; Murray, A.P.; Domini, C.; Werdin-González, J.O. Ultrasound assisted formation of essential oil nanoemulsions: Emerging alternative for *Culex pipiens pipiens* Say (Diptera: Culicidae) and *Plodia interpunctella* Hübner (Lepidoptera: Pyralidae) management. *Ultrason. Sonochem.* **2020**, *61*, 104832. [CrossRef]
50. Louni, M.; Shakarami, J.; Negahban, M. Insecticidal efficacy of nanoemulsion containing *Mentha longifolia* essential oil against *Ephestia kuehniella* (Lepidoptera: Pyralidae). *J. Crop. Prot.* **2018**, *7*, 171–182.
51. Elbadawy, M.A.E.; Azab, M.M.; Shams El Din, A.M.; Radwan, E.M.M. Toxicity of Some Plant Oil Nanoemulsions to Black Cutworm, *Agrotis ipsilon* Hufnagel (Lepidoptera: Noctuidae). *Nanotechnol. Agric. Food Environ.* **2019**, *1*, 1. [CrossRef]
52. Mossa, A.-T.H.; Abdelfatta, N.A.H.; Mohafrash, S.M.M. Nanoemulsion of Camphor (*Eucalyptus globulus*) Essential Oil, Formulation, Characterization and Insecticidal Activity against Wheat Weevil, *Sitophilus granarius*. *Asian J. Crop. Sci.* **2017**, *9*, 50–62. [CrossRef]
53. Balasubramani, S.; Rajendhiran, T.; Moola, A.K.; Diana, R.K.B. Development of nanoemulsion from *Vitex negundo* L. essential oil and their efficacy of antioxidant, antimicrobial and larvicidal activities (*Aedes aegypti* L.). *Environ. Sci. Pollut. Res.* **2017**, *24*, 15125–15133. [CrossRef]
54. Kalaitzaki, A.; Papanikolaou, N.E.; Karamaouna, F.; Dourtoglou, V.; Xenakis, A.; Papadimitriou, V. Biocompatible Colloidal Dispersions as Potential Formulations of Natural Pyrethrins: A Structural and Efficacy Study. *Langmuir* **2015**, *31*, 5722–5730. [CrossRef] [PubMed]
55. Kavallieratos, N.G.; Boukouvala, M.C.; Ntalli, N.; Skourti, A.; Karagianni, E.S.; Nika, E.P.; Kontodimas, D.C.; Cappellacci, L.; Petrelli, R.; Cianfaglione, K.; et al. Effectiveness of eight essential oils against two key stored-product beetles, *Prostephanus truncatus* (Horn) and *Trogoderma granarium* Everts. *Food Chem. Toxicol.* **2020**, *139*, 111255. [CrossRef] [PubMed]
56. Benelli, G.; Pavela, R.; Petrelli, R.; Nzekoue, F.K.; Cappellacci, L.; Lupidi, G.; Quassinti, L.; Bramucci, M.; Sut, S.; Dall'Acqua, S.; et al. Carlina oxide from *Carlina acaulis* root essential oil acts as a potent mosquito larvicide. *Ind. Crops Prod.* **2019**, *137*, 356–366. [CrossRef]
57. Tutin, T.G.; Heywood, V.H.; Burges, N.A.; Moore, D.M.; Valentine, D.H.; Walters, S.M.; Webb, D.A. *Flora Europaea. Volume 4. Plantaginaceae to Compositae (and Rubiaceae)*; Cambridge University Press: Cambridge, UK, 1976. [CrossRef]
58. Pharmacopoeia Bavarica, Monachii. 1822. Available online: https://archive.org/details/pharmacopoeabava00mona/page/n3/mode/2up (accessed on 21 May 2020).
59. Bukowiecki, H.; Furmanó, M.; Sujka, J. Medical herbs. In *Pharmacopoeia Regni Poloniae*; Typographia juxta Novolipium Nro 646: Warsaw, Poland, 1817; Volume 16, pp. 15–53.
60. Pharmacopoeia Universalis, Weimar. 1832. Available online: https://reader.digitale-sammlungen.de/de/fs1/object/display/bsb1028803000009.html (accessed on 21 May 2020).
61. Pharmacopoeia Universalis, Weimar. 1838. Available online: https://reader.digitale-sammlungen.de/de/fs1/object/display/bsb1028803000009.html (accessed on 22 May 2020).
62. Hort, A.S. *Theophrastus: Enquiry into Plants, and Minor Works on Odours and Weather Signs*; Loeb Classical Library 79; Harvard University Press: Cambridge, MA, USA; William Heinemann: London, UK, 1949; Volume 2.
63. Ruellio, I. *Pedanii Dioscoridis Anazarbei, De Medicinali Materia Libri Sex*; Apud Balthazarem Arnolletum: Lugduni, Rome, 1552; pp. 1–828. [CrossRef]
64. Kluk, J.K. *Dykcjonarz Roślinny*; Drukarnia Xięży Pijarów: Warsaw, Poland, 1805.
65. Guarrera, P.M. Food medicine and minor nourishment in the folk traditions of Central Italy (Marche, Abruzzo and Latium). *Fitoterapia* **2003**, *74*, 515–544. [CrossRef]
66. Menale, B.; Amato, G.; Prisco, C.D.; Muoio, R. Traditional uses of plants in North-Western Molise (Central Italy). *Delpinoa* **2006**, *48*, 29–36. [CrossRef]
67. Redzić, S.S. The ecological aspect of ethnobotany and ethnopharmacology of population in Bosnia and Herzegovina. *Coll. Antropol.* **2007**, *31*, 869–890. [PubMed]

68. Strzemski, M.; Wojnicki, K.; Sowa, I.; Wojas-Krawczyk, K.; Krawczyk, P.; Kocjan, R.; Such, J.; Latalski, M.; Wnorowski, A.; Wójciak-Kosior, M. In Vitro Antiproliferative Activity of Extracts of *Carlina acaulis* subsp. *caulescens* and *Carlina acanthifolia* subsp. *utzka*. *Front. Pharmacol.* **2017**, *8*, 371. [CrossRef]
69. Gazzetta Ufficiale. Available online: https://www.gazzettaufficiale.it/eli/gu/2018/09/26/224/sg/pdf (accessed on 27 May 2020).
70. Cousyn, G.; Dalfrà, S.; Scarpa, B.; Geelen, J.; Anton, R.; Serafini, M.; Delmulle, L. Project belfrit: Harmonizing the use of plants in food supplements in the european union: Belgium, France and Italy—A first step. *Eur. Food Feed Law Rev.* **2013**, *8*, 187–196.
71. Pavela, R.; Maggi, F.; Petrelli, R.; Cappellacci, L.; Buccioni, M.; Palmieri, A.; Canale, A.; Benelli, G. Outstanding insecticidal activity and sublethal effects of *Carlina acaulis* root essential oil on the housefly, *Musca domestica*, with insights on its toxicity on human cells. *Food Chem. Toxicol.* **2020**, *136*, 111037. [CrossRef]
72. Vanden Dool, H.; Kratz, P.D. A generalization of the retention index system including linear temperature programmed gas-liquid partition chromatography. *J. Chromatogr.* **1963**, *11*, 463–471. [CrossRef]
73. Rosi Cappellani, M.; Perinelli, D.R.; Pescosolido, L.; Schoubben, A.; Cespi, M.; Cossi, R.; Blasi, P. Injectable nanoemulsions prepared by high pressure homogenization: Processing, sterilization, and size evolution. *Appl. Nanosci. Switz.* **2018**, *8*, 1483–1491. [CrossRef]
74. Alkilani, A.Z.; Hamed, R.; Al-Marabeh, S.; Kamal, A.; Abu-Huwaij, R.; Hamad, I. Nanoemulsion-based film formulation for transdermal delivery of carvedilol. *J. Drug Deliv. Sci. Technol.* **2018**, *46*, 122–128. [CrossRef]
75. Gabel, B. Über eine neue semisynthetische Nahrung für die Raupen des Bekreuzten Traubenwicklers, *Lobesia botrana* Den. et Schiff. (Lepid., Tortricidae). *Anz. Für Schädlingskunde Pflanzenschutz Umweltschutz* **1980**, *53*, 72–74. [CrossRef]
76. Bosch, D.; Rodríguez, M.; Avilla, J. A new bioassay to test insecticide resistance of *Cydia pomonella* (L.) first instar larvae: Results from some field populations of Lleida (Spain). *Pome Fruit Arthropods IOBC/wprs Bulletin.* **2007**, *30*, 195–199.
77. Abbott, W.S. A Method of Computing the Effectiveness of an Insecticide. *J. Econ. Entomol.* **1925**, *18*, 265–267. [CrossRef]
78. Finney, D.J. *Statistical Method in Biological Assay*, 3rd ed; Hodder Arnold: London, UK, 1978.
79. Pavoni, L.; Perinelli, D.R.; Bonacucina, G.; Cespi, M.; Palmieri, G.F. An Overview of Micro-and Nanoemulsions as Vehicles for Essential Oils: Formulation, Preparation and Stability. *Nanomaterials* **2020**, *10*, 135. [CrossRef]
80. Pavela, R.; Pavoni, L.; Bonacucina, G.; Cespi, M.; Kavallieratos, N.G.; Cappellacci, L.; Petrelli, R.; Maggi, F.; Benelli, G. Rationale for developing novel mosquito larvicides based on isofuranodiene microemulsions. *J. Pest Sci.* **2019**, *92*, 909–921. [CrossRef]
81. Pavela, R.; Benelli, G.; Pavoni, L.; Bonacucina, G.; Cespi, M.; Cianfaglione, K.; Bajalan, I.; Morshedloo, M.R.; Lupidi, G.; Romano, D.; et al. Microemulsions for delivery of Apiaceae essential oils—Towards highly effective and eco-friendly mosquito larvicides? *Ind. Crops Prod.* **2019**, *129*, 631–640. [CrossRef]
82. Rao, J.; McClements, D.J. Formation of flavor oil microemulsions, nanoemulsions and emulsions: Influence of composition and preparation method. *J. Agric. Food Chem.* **2011**, *59*, 5026–5035. [CrossRef]
83. Yuan, Y.; Gao, Y.; Zhao, J.; Mao, L. Characterization and stability evaluation of β-carotene nanoemulsions prepared by high pressure homogenization under various emulsifying conditions. *Food Res. Int.* **2008**, *41*, 61–68. [CrossRef]
84. Gupta, A.; Eral, H.B.; Hatton, T.A.; Doyle, P.S. Nanoemulsions: Formation, properties and applications. *Soft Matter.* **2016**, *12*, 2826–2841. [CrossRef] [PubMed]
85. Sadeghi, R.; Etemad, S.G.; Keshavarzi, E.; Haghshenasfard, M. Investigation of alumina nanofluid stability by UV-vis spectrum. *Microfluid. Nanofluidics* **2015**, *18*, 1023–1030. [CrossRef]
86. Ammar, H.O.; Salama, H.A.; Ghorab, M.; Mahmoud, A.A. Nanoemulsion as a potential ophthalmic delivery system for dorzolamide hydrochloride. *AAPS PharmSciTech* **2009**, *10*, 808. [CrossRef] [PubMed]
87. Huang, Q.; Yu, H.; Ru, Q. Bioavailability and delivery of nutraceuticals using nanotechnology. *J. Food Sci.* **2010**, *75*, R50–R57. [CrossRef] [PubMed]
88. Cattaneo, A.M.; Bengtsson, J.M.; Borgonovo, G.; Bassoli, A.; Anfora, G. Response of the European grapevine moth *Lobesia botrana* to somatosensory-active volatiles emitted by the non-host plant *Perilla frutescens*. *Physiol. Entomol.* **2014**, *39*, 229–236. [CrossRef]
89. Katerinopoulos, H.E.; Pagona, G.; Afratis, A.; Stratigakis, N.; Roditakis, N. Composition and insect attracting activity of the Essential oil of *Rosmarinus officinalis*. *J. Chem. Ecol.* **2005**, *31*, 111–122. [CrossRef] [PubMed]

90. Konovalov, D.A. Polyacetylene Compounds of Plants of the Asteraceae Family (Review). *Pharm. Chem. J.* **2014**, *48*, 613–631. [CrossRef]
91. Czyzewska, M.M.; Chrobok, L.; Kania, A.; Jatczak, M.; Pollastro, F.; Appendino, G.; Mozrzymas, J.W. Dietary Acetylenic Oxylipin Falcarinol Differentially Modulates GABAA Receptors. *J. Nat. Prod.* **2014**, *77*, 2671–2677. [CrossRef]
92. Pavela, R. Essential oils for the development of eco-friendly mosquito larvicides: A review. *Ind. Crops Prod.* **2015**, *76*, 174–187. [CrossRef]
93. Pavela, R.; Maggi, F.; Iannarelli, R.; Benelli, G. Plant extracts for developing mosquito larvicides: From laboratory to the field, with insights on the modes of action. *Acta Trop.* **2019**, *193*, 236–271. [CrossRef]
94. Isman, M.B. Botanical Insecticides in the Twenty-First Century—Fulfilling Their Promise? *Annu. Rev. Entomol.* **2019**, *65*, 233–249. [CrossRef] [PubMed]
95. Rizzo, R.; Lo Verde, G.; Sinacori, M.; Maggi, F.; Cappellacci, L.; Petrelli, R.; Vittori, S.; Morshedloo, M.R.; Fofie, N.G.B.Y.; Benelli, G. Developing green insecticides to manage olive fruit flies? Ingestion toxicity of four essential oils in protein baits on *Bactrocera oleae*. *Ind. Crops Prod.* **2020**, *143*, 111884. [CrossRef]

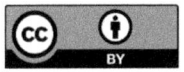

© 2020 by the authors. Licensee MDPI, Basel, Switzerland. This article is an open access article distributed under the terms and conditions of the Creative Commons Attribution (CC BY) license (http://creativecommons.org/licenses/by/4.0/).

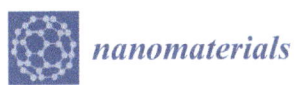

Article

Tunable Terahertz Metamaterial with Electromagnetically Induced Transparency Characteristic for Sensing Application

Jitong Zhong, Xiaocan Xu and Yu-Sheng Lin *

School of Electronics and Information Technology, Sun Yat-Sen University, Guangzhou 510006, China; zhongjt5@mail2.sysu.edu.cn (J.Z.); xuxc5@mail2.sysu.edu.cn (X.X.)
* Correspondence: linyoush@mail.sysu.edu.cn

Abstract: We present and demonstrate a MEMS-based tunable terahertz metamaterial (TTM) composed of inner triadius and outer electric split-ring resonator (eSRR) structures. With the aim to explore the electromagnetic responses of TTM device, different geometrical parameters are compared and discussed to optimize the suitable TTM design, including the length, radius, and height of TTM device. The height of triadius structure could be changed by using MEMS technique to perform active tunability. TTM shows the polarization-dependent and electromagnetic induced transparency (EIT) characteristics owing to the eSRR configuration. The electromagnetic responses of TTM exhibit tunable characteristics in resonance, polarization-dependent, and electromagnetically induced transparency (EIT). By properly tailoring the length and height of the inner triadius structure and the radius of the outer eSRR structure, the corresponding resonance tuning range reaches 0.32 THz. In addition to the above optical characteristics of TTM, we further investigate its potential application in a refraction index sensor. TTM is exposed on the surrounding ambient with different refraction indexes. The corresponding key sensing performances, such as figure of merit (FOM), sensitivity (S), and quality factor (Q-factor) values, are calculated and discussed, respectively. The calculated sensitivity of TTM is 0.379 THz/RIU, while the average values of Q-factor and FOM are 66.01 and 63.83, respectively. These characteristics indicate that the presented MEMS-based TTM device could be widely used in tunable filters, perfect absorbers, high-efficient environmental sensors, and optical switches applications for THz-wave optoelectronics.

Keywords: electromechanically; tunability; metamaterials; multi-functionalities; terahertz; refraction index sensor

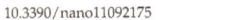

Citation: Zhong, J.; Xu, X.; Lin, Y.-S. Tunable Terahertz Metamaterial with Electromagnetically Induced Transparency Characteristic for Sensing Application. *Nanomaterials* 2021, *11*, 2175. https://doi.org/10.3390/nano11092175

Academic Editor: Giovanni Benelli

Received: 6 July 2021
Accepted: 28 July 2021
Published: 25 August 2021

Publisher's Note: MDPI stays neutral with regard to jurisdictional claims in published maps and institutional affiliations.

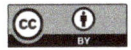

Copyright: © 2021 by the authors. Licensee MDPI, Basel, Switzerland. This article is an open access article distributed under the terms and conditions of the Creative Commons Attribution (CC BY) license (https://creativecommons.org/licenses/by/4.0/).

1. Introduction

Metamaterials are regarded as artificial materials that are remain undiscovered in the natural environment [1–3]. Due to their extraordinary properties, metamaterials are becoming an emerging field in physics, chemical, engineering, and electrics subjects. In the recent years, there have been many investigations and reports in various potential applications of metamaterials, such as cloaking devices, high-sensitive environment sensors, perfect absorbers, security screening, tunable ultrahigh-speed filters, imaging devices, high-efficient light emitters, and non-destructive testing [3–10]. Metamaterials show many unique electromagnetic properties including field enhancement [11,12], negative refraction index [13], artificial magnetism [14], electromagnetically induced transparency (EIT) [15], and so on. By properly tailoring the geometric parameters, metamaterials are able to be easily operated in a wide spectrum range that includes terahertz (THz), infrared (IR), and visible light [16–26]. Among the whole electromagnetic spectra, THz wave is the transition spectrum that usually occupies the spectrum in the frequency range from 0.1 THz to 10 THz, which is between the IR and microwave wavelengths. Since that metamaterial has great and ultra-sensitive electromagnetic response in the THz frequency range, THz metamaterial has become an emerging field during the recent years. One of the most used typical configurations of THz metamaterial is a split-ring resonator (SRR), which is commonly a ring with a split. It was theoretically proposed in 1999 for the first time and experimentally verified in 2000. Since then, many derivative designs were investigated and demonstrated based on SRR, such as the complementary SRR (cSRR) [27], V-shaped SRR [28], U-shaped SRR [29], electric SRR (eSRR) [30,31], and three-dimensional SRR (3D SRR) [32,33], etc. However, when the metamaterial structure is fabricated on the traditional solid substrates, the resonant frequencies of metamaterial are usually unable to be tuned, which means that these designs can only absorb or filter certain electromagnetic spectra in a passive manner. Aiming to improve the flexibility and to enhance the electromagnetic response of the THz metamaterial, many literature reports focusing on tuning mechanisms were reported, such as ferroelectric material [34,35], laser pumping [36,37], electrostatic force [38,39], thermal annealing [40,41], liquid crystal [42], semiconductor material [43], and so on. In addition, micro-/nano-electro-mechanical systems (MEMS/NEMS) technologies can easily realize mechanical manipulation in micro-scale or nano-scale and, as a result, can hugely improve flexibility and enhance the electromagnetic response of MEMS-based metamaterial in the THz frequency range. There have been many reports on MEMS devices with different tuning mechanisms, such as the electrothermal actuator, electrostatic actuator, piezoelectric actuator, electromagnetic actuator [44–47], etc.

In this study, we propose and demonstrate a tunable terahertz metamaterial (TTM) based on the MEMS technology in the THz frequency range. This TTM structure is composed of an inner Au layer, which is called a triadius structure, and an outer Au layer, which is called a eSRR structure. The whole structure is fabricated on Si substrate. The inner triadius structures are connected to the MEMS-based electrothermal actuator (ETA). By driving different dc bias voltages, the height between the triadius and eSRR structures can be changed and, therefore, exhibit high flexibility. The geometrical dimensions of the proposed TTM are optimized, including the length and height of inner triadius structure and the radius of outer eSRR structure. The field strengths distributions in this study, including the electric (E) and magnetic (H) fields of the triadius structure, eSRR structure, and TTM structure, will be analyzed and discussed, respectively. In addition, in order to investigate the potential applications of TTM in the environmental sensing application, the key sensing performances of TTM, such as figure of merit (FOM), sensitivity (S), and quality factor (Q-factor), will be calculated and discussed, respectively. Additionally, while exposed on different-refraction-index (n value) environment, TTM shows highly linear sensitivity in terms of the n values. These unique electromagnetic characteristics indicate that the TTM structure can be widely used in THz-range application fields, such as filters, switches, and high-efficient environment sensors including gas sensors, biosensors, chemical sensors, etc.

2. Design and Method

The schematic drawings of MEMS-based TTM and TTM unit cell are shown in Figure 1a,b, respectively. TTM is composed of the triadius and eSRR structures. A 300 nm thick Au layer is used in TTM. The inner triadius structures are connected to MEMS-based electrothermal actuator (ETA), which could exhibit high flexibility by driving different dc bias voltages to bend downwards. Figure 1c shows the geometrical denotations of the TTM unit cell, including metal length (L), radius of eSRR (R), and height between inner triadius and outer eSRR structures (h). The metal linewidth and gap of the inner triadius and outer eSRR structures are 5 μm. Figure 1d plots the relationship of driving voltages and displacements of MEMS-based TTM. The inserted images of Figure 1d are the geometrical dimensions of ETA. Due to the different thermal expansion coefficients between different materials, the cantilevers would be upward-bending after the release process in fabrication. Therefore, by driving different dc bias voltages on ETAs, the reconfiguration of MEMS-based TTM was proposed in order to compare and discuss different h values. The deformation in the free end of ETA is inversely related to applied voltage. In order to actuate the TTM unit cell for bending downwards, a driving voltage with a maximum value of 0.45 V would be induced on the TTM device. The inserted images include the inner triadius structure on ETA without and with a driving voltage of 0.45 V, respectively. The initial height is h = 2.46 µm when the MEMS-based TTM is released, while h value will be bent to 0 µm when the driving voltage increases to 0.45 V. It is clear that the proposed MEMS-based TTM could be actively actuated to tune the resonance by bending the cantilevers downwards.

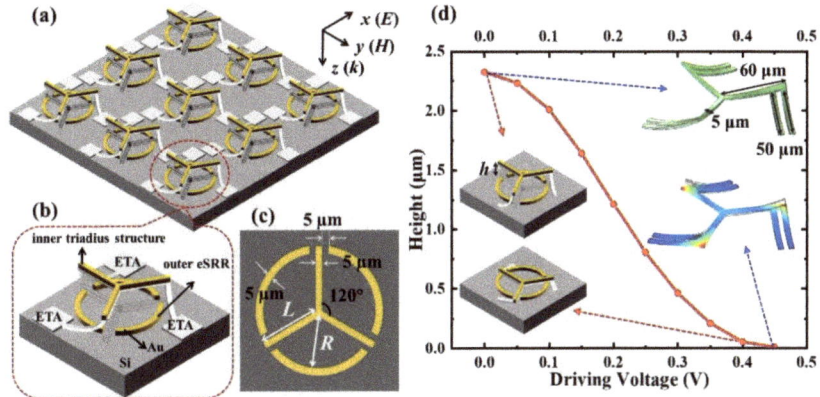

Figure 1. Schematic drawing of (**a**) MEMS-based TTM and (**b**) unit cell in detail. (**c**) Top view of TTM unit cell and the corresponding geometrical denotations. (**d**) Relationship of driving voltages and elevating heights (h) of TTM with ETA. Inserted images are the ETA simulations.

The optical properties of the proposed TTM device are simulated by using Lumerical Solution's finite difference time domain (FDTD) based simulations. Here, we define TE mode when the polarization angle equals to 0° and TM mode when the polarization angle equals to 90°. The propagation direction of incident light is set to be perpendicular to the x-y plane in the numerical simulations. Periodic boundary conditions are also adopted in the x-axis and y-axis directions and perfectly matched layer (PML) boundaries conditions are assumed in the z-axis direction. The transmission spectra (T) are calculated by monitor set on below of device. In these configurations, Si material serves as the substrate with the tailored Au layer atop. The permittivity values of Au and Si materials in the mid-IR wavelength range are calculated according to the Drude–Lorentz model [48,49].

3. Results and Discussion

The transmission spectra of the triadius structure in TE and TM modes with different L values are shown in Figure 2, respectively. This triadius structure shows polarization-dependent characteristics. For example, when L = 47.5 µm, the TE and TM resonances are at 0.58 THz. With L value decreasing by 5 µm steps from 47.5 µm to 32.5 µm, both TE and TM resonances are increased by 0.16 THz, (from 0.58 THz to 0.74 THz). As plotted in Figure 3, the field strength distributions (E-fields and H-fields) of the triadius structure possess a L value of 42.5 µm when monitored at 0.58 THz in TE and TM modes, respectively. The E-field strengths are focused on the end of the triadius structure, while the H-field strengths are concentrated along the contour of the triadius structure.

The transmission spectra with different R values of eSRR structure in TE and TM modes are shown in Figure 4a,b, respectively. In Figure 4a, eSRR shows the EIT characteristic at 0.60 THz with R = 45 µm. The EIT resonance is shifted to 0.68 THz and the R value decreased to 40 µm. The shifting range of EIT resonance is 0.08 THz. This EIT resonance gradually vanishes by continuously decreasing R value to 30 µm. By decreasing R value in 5 µm steps (gradually from 45 µm to 30 µm), the resonances are blue-shifted with a shifting range of 0.40 THz (from 0.58 THz with R = 45 µm to 0.98 THz with R = 30 µm). On the other hand, in the TM mode, by decreasing R value in 5 µm steps (gradually from 45 µm to 30 µm), the resonances are modified with a modifying range of 0.32 THz (from 0.67 THz with R = 45 µm to 0.99 THz with R = 30 µm). According to the results mentioned above, eSRR exhibits polarization-dependent characteristics. Figure 5 plots the field strengths distributions (E- and H-fields) of eSRR with a R value of 40 µm in TE and TM modes, respectively. In TE mode, the monitors of field distributions are set as 0.67 THz, 0.68 THz, and 0.70 TH, while it is set as 0.74 THz in TM mode. It can be observed in Figure 5a–c that the E-field strengths are focused on the ends of arc-shape of eSRR in order to generate the electric quadrupole, six-polar, and dipolar modes at 0.67 THz, 0.68 THz, and 0.70 THz, respectively. Meanwhile, the E-field strengths of TM resonance are focused on the on the ends of the arc-shape of eSRR, which is the electric quadrupole mode as shown in Figure 5d. The corresponding H-field strengths of eSRR in TE and TM modes are shown in Figure 5e–h for the electric quadrupole, six-polar, and dipolar modes at 0.67 THz, 0.68 THz, and 0.70 THz for TE resonance and electric quadrupole mode at 0.74 THz for TM resonance, respectively.

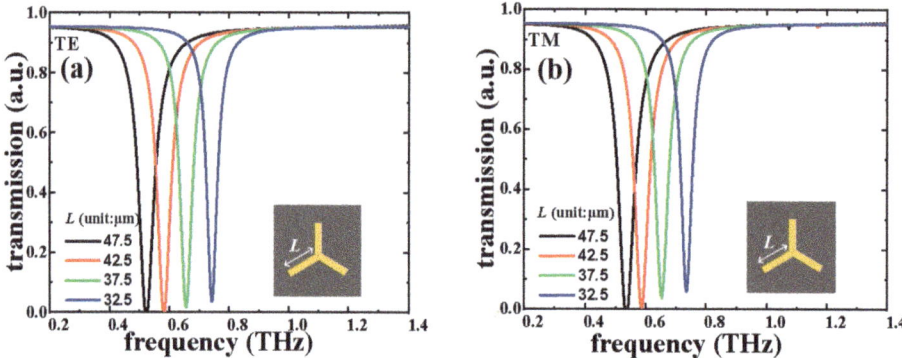

Figure 2. Electromagnetic responses of the triadius structure by changing the L parameter in (**a**) TE and (**b**) TM modes.

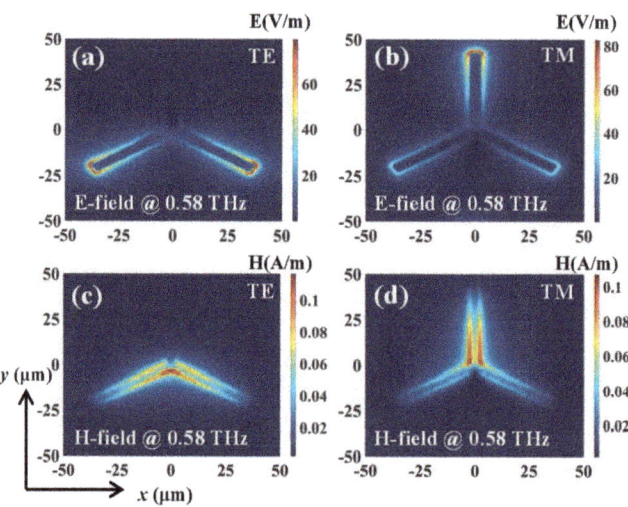

Figure 3. Field distributions of the triadius structure with L = 42.5 µm in TE and TM modes. (**a**) and (**b**) are E-field distributions. (**c**) and (**d**) are H-field distributions.

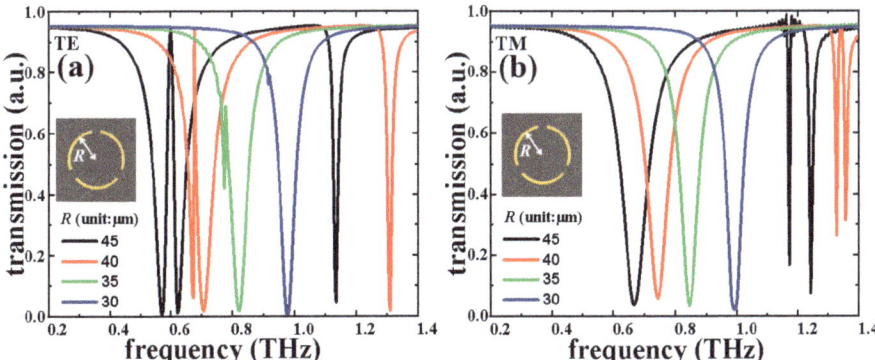

Figure 4. Electromagnetic responses of eSRR by changing the R parameter in (**a**) TE and (**b**) TM modes.

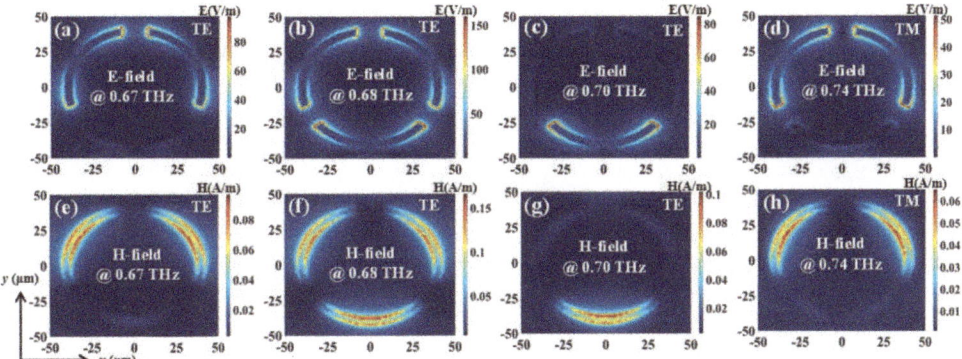

Figure 5. Field distributions of eSRR with R = 40 µm in TE and TM modes. (**a–d**) are E-field distributions. (**e–h**) are H-field distributions.

The transmission spectra of TTM with different R values in TE and TM modes with a constant L value of 47.5 µm are shown in Figure 6a,b, respectively. The resonances are superimposed from the resonances of the triadius and eSRR structures. For example, when R = 45 µm, the second TE resonance is at 0.66 THz while the second TM resonance is at 0.70 THz, respectively. By decreasing the R value in 5 µm steps (from 45 µm to 30 µm), the second TE resonance is increased to 0.32 THz (from 0.66 THz with R = 45 µm to 0.98 THz with R = 30 µm), while the second TM resonance is increased to 0.30 THz (from 0.70 THz for R = 45 µm to 1.00 THz for R = 30 µm). Meanwhile, since the L value is kept as constant at 47.5 µm, the first TE and TM resonances influenced by the triadius structure almost remain unchanged. TTM shows the EIT characteristic at 0.60 THz with R = 45 µm in TE mode as shown in Figure 6a. The EIT resonance is shifted to 0.67 THz with the R value decreased to 40 µm. The shifting range of EIT resonance is 0.07 THz. This EIT resonance gradually vanishes by continuously decreasing the R value to 30 µm. The field strengths distributions (E-fields and H-fields) of TTM with L value of 47.5 µm and R value of 40 µm in TE and TM modes are plotted in Figure 7, respectively. In TE mode, the monitors of field distributions are set at 0.53 THz, 0.67 THz, and 0.73 THz, while in TM mode they are set at 0.54 THz and 0.78 THz. As observed in Figures 7a–c and 7g–h, the E-field strengths are focused on the end of the triadius structure as well as the ends of the arc-shape of eSRR for both TE and TM resonances, respectively. Meanwhile, plotted in Figures 7d–f and 7i–j are the corresponding H-field distributions of TTM in TE and TM modes (0.53 THz, 0.67 THz, and 0.73 THz for TE resonances; 0.54 THz and 0.78 THz for TM resonances), respectively.

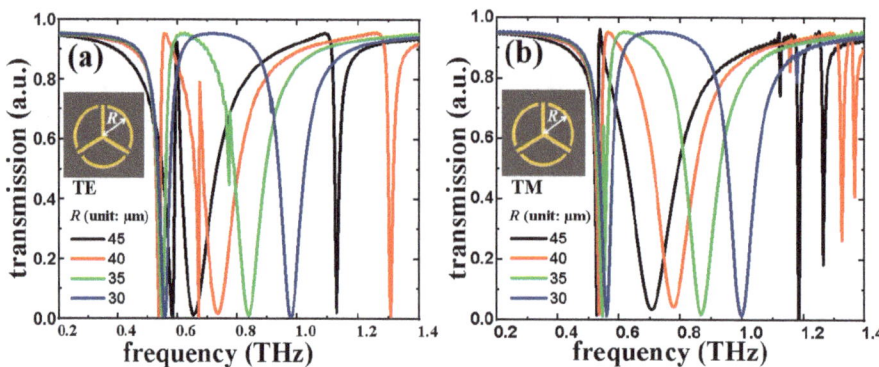

Figure 6. Electromagnetic responses of TTM by changing the *R* parameter in (**a**) TE and (**b**) TM modes under the condition of *L* = 47.5 μm.

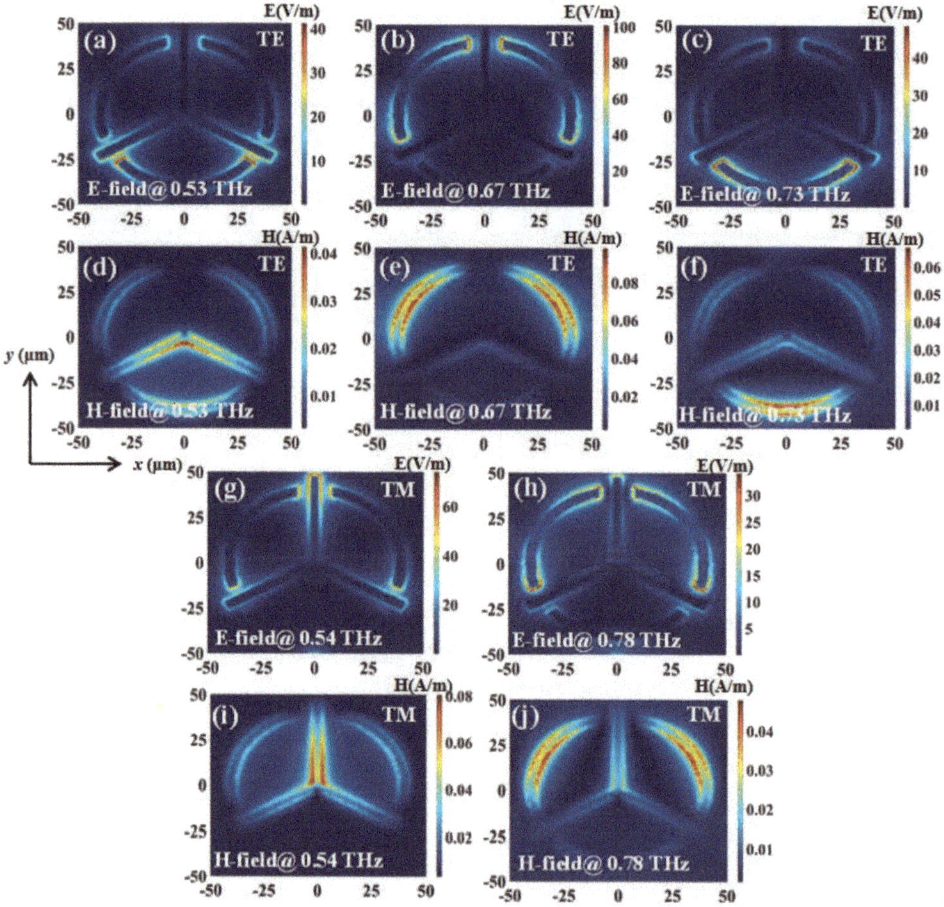

Figure 7. Field distributions of TTM with *L* = 47.5 μm and *R* = 40 μm in TE and TM modes. (**a–c,g,h**) are E-field distributions. (**d–f,i,j**) are H-field distributions.

The transmission spectra of TTM structure with different h values in TE and TM modes with a constant L value of 47.5 μm and a constant R value of 40 μm are plotted in Figure 8. The resonances are superimposed from the resonances of the triadius and eSRR structures. For example, when h = 0 μm, the first TE resonance is at 0.49 THz while the first TM resonance is at 0.51 THz, respectively. By increasing the h value from 0 μm to 3 μm, the first TE resonance is increased to 0.09 THz (from 0.49 THz for h = 0 μm to 0.58 THz for h = 3 μm), while the first TM resonance is increased to 0.07 THz (from 0.51 THz for h = 0 μm to 0.58 THz for h = 3 μm). Meanwhile, since the height of the eSRR structure is kept constant at 0 μm and the R value is kept constant at 40 μm, the second TE and TM resonances influenced by eSRR structure almost remain unchanged. Particularly, in TE mode, TTM with R = 40 μm shows the EIT characteristic at 0.67 THz. The field strengths distributions (E-fields and H-fields) of TTM with the L value of 47.5 μm, R value of 40 μm, and h value of 1 μm in TE and TM modes are plotted in Figure 7, respectively. In TE mode, the monitors of field distributions are set at 0.54 THz, 0.67 THz, and 0.73 THz, while in TM mode they are set at 0.54 THz and 0.78 THz. In Figures 9a–c and 9g–h, the E-field strengths are focused on the end of the triadius structure as well as the ends of the arc-shape of eSRR for TE and TM resonances, respectively. Meanwhile, the corresponding H-field distributions of TTM in TE and TM modes are plotted in Figures 9d–f and 9i–j, respectively.

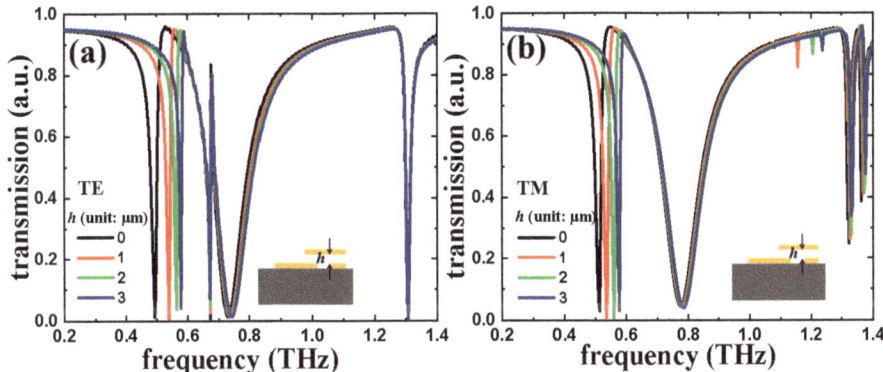

Figure 8. Electromagnetic responses of TTM by changing the h parameter in (**a**) TE and (**b**) TM modes.

In order to further explore the potential applications of the proposed TTM device in environmental sensing, the key sensing performances of TTM, such as figure of merit (FOM), sensitivity (S), and quality factor (Q-factor), are investigated. In this study, TTM with constant geometrical parameters (L = 47.5 μm, R = 40 μm, and h = 0 μm) is exposed on the surrounding ambient with different refraction indexes (n values). Figure 10a,b shows the trends of sensitivities between TE and TM resonances and n values, respectively. They are quite linear. Here, we define the corresponding resonances in TE and TM modes and the sensitivities as ω_1, ω_2, ω_3, and $S = \Delta f/\Delta n$, respectively. The Δf is the shift of resonant frequency and Δn is the change of n value. In TE mode, the calculated S at ω_1, ω_2, and ω_3 are 0.138 THz/RIU, 0.21 THz/RIU, and 0.379 THz/RIU, respectively. It is obvious that the third resonance (ω_3) is more sensitive to the n value than the others. In TM mode, the corresponding S values at three resonances are 0.15 THz/RIU, 0.223 THz/RIU, and 0.373 THz/RIU, respectively. Obviously, these results indicate that the third resonance is more sensitive to the n value as well. The definition of Q-factor is that $Q = f_r/\text{FWHM}$ and FOM are defined as FOM = $(1 - A_r) \times Q$ [50], where f_r is the frequency of resonance and A_r is the corresponding transmission amplitudes, respectively. The calculated Q-factors and FOMs values at different TE and TM resonances are plotted in Figure 10c,d, respectively. Table 1 is a summary table of the corresponding Q-factors and FOMs values. Let us take the third TE resonance (TE: ω_3, green line) as an example, then the maximum, minimum, and average values of the calculated Q-factors are 72.47, 59.91, and 66.01, respectively, while the corresponding calculated FOMs values are 71.33, 56.49, and 63.83, respectively. The sensing performances of this design are better than those reported in literature reports [9,15,51] as summarized in Table 2. Therefore, the proposed MEMS-based TTM device could be suitably used in environment sensing fields, such as gas sensing, bio-sensing, and chemical sensing, etc.

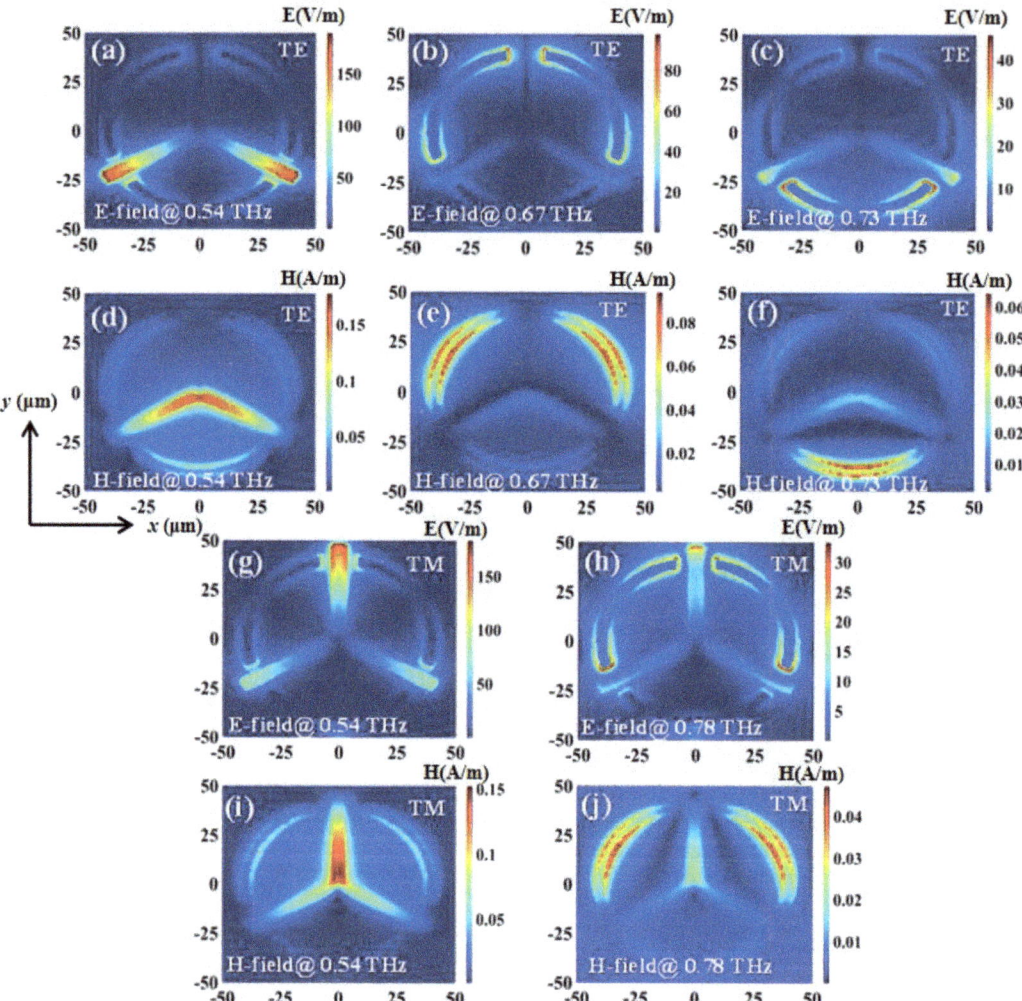

Figure 9. Field distributions of TTM with $h = 1$ µm in TE and TM modes. (**a**–**c**,**g**,**h**) are E-field distributions. (**d**–**f**,**i**,**j**) are H-field distributions.

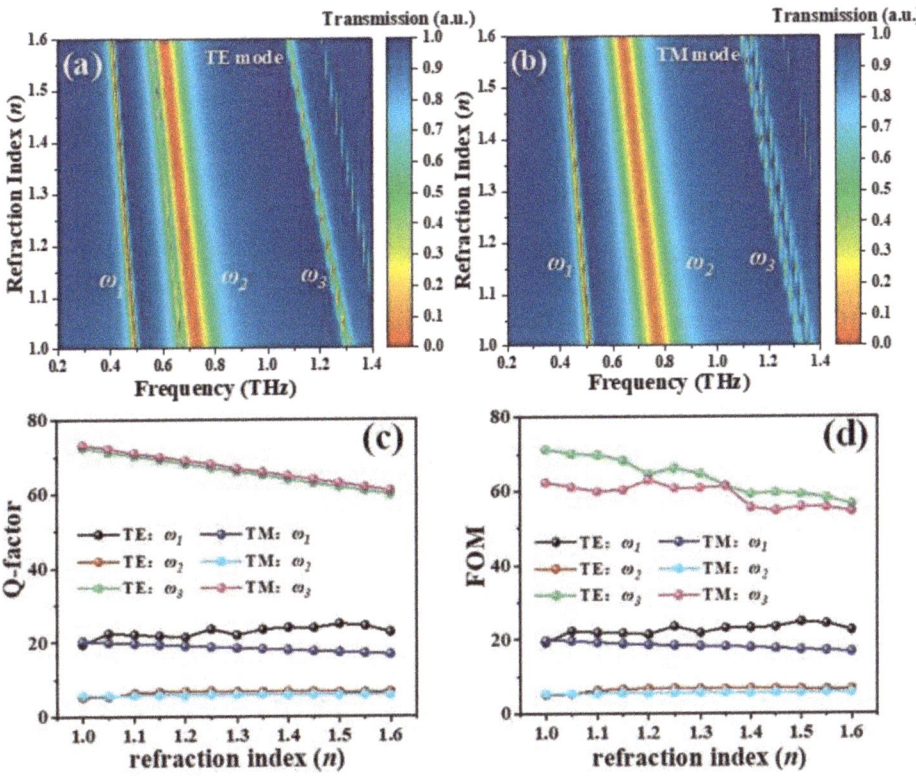

Figure 10. Electromagnetic responses of the TTM exposed on the surrounding ambient with different refraction index (n) in (**a**) TE and (**b**) TM modes, where L, R, and h parameters are kept as constants at 47.5 μm, 40 μm, and 0 μm, respectively. (**c**,**d**) are the Q-factors and FOMs of TTM in TE and TM modes, respectively.

Table 1. Summaries of Q-factors and FOMs of TTM.

Resonance	Q-Factor			FOM		
	Max.	Min.	Ave.	Max.	Min.	Ave.
TE: ω_1	24.89	19.49	22.76	24.78	19.22	22.54
TE: ω_2	6.94	5.19	6.50	6.87	5.12	6.44
TE: ω_3	72.47	59.91	66.01	71.33	56.49	63.83
TM: ω_1	20.35	16.78	18.50	19.72	16.69	18.25
TM: ω_2	6.11	5.64	5.90	5.84	5.40	5.66
TM: ω_3	73.27	60.91	62.10	62.33	54.51	58.92

Table 2. The comparison of sensing performances in this study and literature reports.

	ω_1	ω_2	ω_3	Reference
Sensitivity (S)	54.18 GHz/RIU	119.2 GHz/RIU	139.2 GHz/RIU	[15]
Sensitivity (S)	128 GHz/RIU	-	-	[51]
Sensitivity (S)	138 GHz/RIU	210 GHz/RIU	379 GHz/RIU	This study
Quality-factor (Max.)	11.6	-	-	[9]

Table 2. Cont.

	ω_1	ω_2	ω_3	Reference
Quality-factor (Max.)	24.89	6.94	72.47	This study
FOM (Max.)	2.30	-	-	[9]
FOM (Max.)	24.78	6.87	71.33	This study

4. Conclusions

In conclusion, a reshaping TTM structure is presented and it is composed of triadius and eSRR structures. By tailoring the geometrical parameters of TTM, such as the length (L value) and height (h value) of the inner triadius structure and the radius (R value) of the outer eSRR structure, the corresponding electromagnetic behavior exhibits polarization-dependent, tunable bandwidth, electro-magnetically induced transparency (EIT), and large resonance-tuning-range characteristics. The variation of the L value causes the resonance blue-shift with a frequency range of 0.16 THz. While the variation of the R value shows that the transmission bandwidths could be modified to possess EIT characteristics. The variation of the h value shows that the resonance could be tuned 0.09 THz. In addition, by changing the surrounding refraction index (n value), MEMS-based TTM shows ultrahigh sensitivity to the surrounding environment. In TE mode, the calculated sensitivity value reaches 0.379 THz/RIU at most, the maximum Q-factor is 72.47, and the maximum FOM is 71.33. In TM mode, the calculated sensitivity value reaches 0.373 THz/RIU, the maximum Q-factor is 73.27, and the maximum FOM is 62.33. These results indicate that the presented MEMS-based TTM has great characteristics and great application potential for high-flexibility tunable filter, perfect absorber, imaging device, optical detecting, environment sensor, and switch applications in the THz frequency range.

Author Contributions: Conceptualization, Y.-S.L.; methodology, J.Z.; software, J.Z.; validation, J.Z., X.X. and Y.-S.L.; formal analysis, J.Z.; investigation, J.Z.; resources, Y.-S.L.; data curation, J.Z. and X.X.; writing—original draft preparation, J.Z.; writing—review and editing, Y.-S.L.; visualization, J.Z. and Y.-S.L.; supervision, Y.-S.L.; project administration, Y.-S.L.; funding acquisition, Y.-S.L. All authors have read and agreed to the published version of the manuscript.

Funding: This research was funded by the financial support from the Natural Science Foundation of Basic and Applied Foundation of Guangdong Province (2021A1515012217), National Key Research and Development Program of China (2019YFA0705004), and National Natural Science Foundation of China (11690031).

Institutional Review Board Statement: Not applicable.

Informed Consent Statement: Informed consent was obtained from all subjects involved in the study.

Data Availability Statement: No new data were created or analyzed in this study. Data sharing is not applicable to this article.

Acknowledgments: The authors acknowledge the financial support from the Natural Science Foundation of Basic and Applied Foundation of Guangdong Province (2021A1515012217), National Key Research and Development Program of China (2019YFA0705004), National Natural Science Foundation of China (11690031), and the State Key Laboratory of Optoelectronic Materials and Technologies of Sun Yat-Sen University for the use of experimental equipment.

Conflicts of Interest: The authors declare no conflict of interest.

References

1. Kabashin, A.V.; Evans, P.; Pastkovsky, S.; Hendren, W.; Wurtz, G.A.; Atkinson, R.; Pollard, R.; Podolskiy, V.A.; Zayats, A.V. Plasmonic nanorod metamaterials for biosensing. *Nat. Mater.* **2009**, *8*, 867–871. [CrossRef]
2. Sreekanth, K.V.; Alapan, Y.; ElKabbash, M.; Ilker, E.; Hinczewski, M.; Gurkan, U.A.; de Luca, A.; Strangi, G. Extreme sensitivity biosensing platform based on hyperbolic metamaterials. *Nat. Mater.* **2016**, *15*, 621–627. [CrossRef]
3. Xu, Z.; Lin, Y.-S. A stretchable terahertz parabolic-shaped metamaterial. *Adv. Opt. Mater.* **2019**, *7*, 1900379. [CrossRef]

4. Chen, H.T.; Padilla, W.J.; Zide, J.M.O.; Gossard, A.C.; Taylor, A.J.; Averitt, R.D. Active terahertz metamaterial devices. *Nature* **2006**, *444*, 597–600. [CrossRef] [PubMed]
5. Choi, M.; Lee, S.H.; Kim, Y.; Kang, S.B.; Shin, J.; Kwak, M.H.; Kang, K.Y.; Lee, Y.H.; Park, N.; Min, B. A terahertz metamaterial with unnaturally high refractive index. *Nature* **2011**, *470*, 369–373. [CrossRef]
6. Han, Y.; Lin, J.; Lin, Y.-S. Tunable Metamaterial-Based Silicon Waveguide. *Opt. Lett.* **2020**, *45*, 6619–6622. [CrossRef] [PubMed]
7. Lu, F.; Ou, H.; Lin, Y.-S. Reconfigurable Terahertz Switch Using Flexible L-shaped Metamaterial. *Opt. Lett.* **2020**, *45*, 6482–6485. [CrossRef] [PubMed]
8. Xu, R.; Lin, Y.-S. Tunable Infrared Metamaterial Emitter for Gas Sensing Application. *Nanomaterials* **2020**, *10*, 1442. [CrossRef]
9. Xu, R.; Lin, Y.-S. Reconfigurable Multiband Terahertz Metamaterial Using Triple-Cantilevers Resonator Array. *IEEE J. Microelectromechanical Syst.* **2020**, *29*, 1167–1172. [CrossRef]
10. Yang, W.; Lin, Y.-S. Tunable metamaterial filter for optical communication in the terahertz frequency range. *Opt. Express* **2020**, *28*, 17620–17629. [CrossRef]
11. Zhan, S.; Wu, X.; Tan, C.; Xiong, J.; Hu, S.; Hu, J.; Wu, S.; Gao, Y.; Liu, Y. Enhanced upconversion based on the ultrahigh local field enhancement in a multilayered UCNPs-metamaterial composite system. *J. Alloy. Compd. J.* **2018**, *735*, 372–376. [CrossRef]
12. Kozina, M.; Pancaldi, M.; Bernhard, C.; Driel, T.V.; Glownia, J.M.; Marsik, P.; Radovic, M.; Vaz, C.A.F.; Zhu, D.; Bonetti, S.; et al. Local terahertz field enhancement for time-resolved X-ray diffraction. *Appl. Phys. Lett.* **2017**, *110*, 081106. [CrossRef]
13. Wong, Z.; Wang, Y.; O'Brien, K.; Rho, J.; Yin, X.; Zhang, S.; Fang, N.; Yen, T.J.; Zhang, X. Optical and acoustic metamaterials: Superlens, negative refractive index and invisibility cloak. *J. Opt.* **2017**, *19*, 084007. [CrossRef]
14. Lannebere, S.; Campione, S.; Aradian, A.; Albani, M.; Capolino, F. Artificial magnetism at terahertz frequencies from three-dimensional lattices of TiO_2 microspheres accounting for spatial dispersion and magnetoelectric coupling. *J. Opt. Soc. Am. B* **2014**, *31*, 1078–1086. [CrossRef]
15. Zheng, D.; Lin, Y.-S. Tunable dual-split-disk resonator with electromagnetically induced transparency characteristic. *Adv. Mater. Technol.* **2020**, *5*, 202000584. [CrossRef]
16. Lin, Y.-S.; Xu, Z. Reconfigurable Metamaterials for Optoelectronic Applications. *Int. J. Optomechatronics* **2020**, *14*, 78–93. [CrossRef]
17. Ou, H.; Lu, F.; Xu, Z.; Lin, Y.-S. Terahertz metamaterial with multiple resonances for biosensing application. *Nanomaterials* **2020**, *10*, 1038. [CrossRef] [PubMed]
18. Xu, Z.; Lin, Z.; Cheng, S.; Lin, Y.-S. Reconfigurable and tunable Terahertz wrench-shape metamaterial performing programmable characteristic. *Opt. Lett.* **2019**, *44*, 3944–3947. [CrossRef] [PubMed]
19. Xu, T.; Xu, X.; Lin, Y.-S. Tunable Terahertz Free Spectra Range Using Electric Split-Ring Metamaterial. *J. Microelectromechanical Syst. J.* **2021**, *30*, 309–314. [CrossRef]
20. Zhu, F.; Lin, Y.-S. Programmable multidigit metamaterial using terahertz electric split-ring resonator. *Opt. Laser Technol.* **2021**, *134*, 106635. [CrossRef]
21. Ferraro, A.; Zografopoulos, D.C.; Caputo, R.; Beccherelli, R. Periodical Elements as Low-Cost Building Blocks for Tunable Terahert Filters. *IEEE Photon. Technol. Lett.* **2016**, *28*, 2459–2462. [CrossRef]
22. Nemec, H.; Duvillaret, L.; Garet, F.; Kuzel, P.; Xavier, P.; Richard, J.; Rauly, D. Thermally tunable filter for terahertz range based on a one-dimensional photonic crystal with a defect. *J. Appl. Phys.* **2004**, *96*, 4072–4075. [CrossRef]
23. Ferraro, A.; Zografopoulos, D.C.; Caputo, R.; Beccherelli, R. Angle-resolved and polarization-dependent investigation of cross-shaped frequency-selective surface terahertz filters. *Appl. Phys. Lett.* **2017**, *110*, 141107. [CrossRef]
24. Pavia, J.; Souto, N.; Ribeiro, M.A. Design of a Reconfigurable THz Filter Based on Metamaterial Wire Resonators with Applications on Sensor Devices. *Photonics* **2020**, *7*, 7030048. [CrossRef]
25. Xu, R.; Lin, Y.-S. Characterizations of reconfigurable infrared metamaterial absorbers. *Opt. Lett.* **2018**, *43*, 4783–4786. [CrossRef] [PubMed]
26. Xu, R.; Lin, Y.-S. Flexible and Controllable Metadevice Using Self-Assembly MEMS Actuator. *Nano Lett.* **2021**, *21*, 3205–3210. [CrossRef] [PubMed]
27. Zhan, F.; Lin, Y.-S. Tunable Multiresonance Using Complementary Circular Metamaterial. *Opt. Lett.* **2020**, *45*, 3633–3636. [CrossRef] [PubMed]
28. Kishor, K.; Baitha, M.N.; Sinha, R.K.; Labirl, B. Tunable negative refractive index metamaterial from V-shaped SRR structure: Fabrication and characterization. *J. Opt. Soc. Am. B* **2014**, *31*, 1410–1414. [CrossRef]
29. Xu, X.; Xu, R.; Lin, Y.-S. Tunable Terahertz Double Split-Ring Metamaterial with Polarization-Sensitive Characteristic. *Opt. Laser Technol.* **2021**, *141*, 107103. [CrossRef]
30. Hu, F.; Xu, N.; Wang, W.; Wang, Y.; Zhang, W.; Han, J.; Zhang, W. A dynamically tunable terahertz metamaterial absorber based on an electrostatic MEMS actuator and electrical dipole resonator array. *J. Micromechanics Microengineering* **2016**, *26*, 025006. [CrossRef]
31. Hu, F.; Qian, Y.; Li, Z.; Niu, J.; Nie, K.; Xiong, X.; Zhang, W.; Peng, Z. Design of a tunable terahertz narrowband metamaterial absorber based on an electrostatically actuated MEMS cantilever and split ring resonator array. *J. Opt.* **2013**, *15*, 055101. [CrossRef]
32. Liu, N.; Guo, H.; Fu, L.; Kaiser, S.; Schweizer, H.; Giessen, H. Three-dimensional photonic metamaterials at optical frequencies. *Nat. Mater.* **2008**, *7*, 31–37. [CrossRef]
33. Chen, C.; Ishikawa, A.; Tand, Y.H.; Shiao, M.H.; Tsai, D.P.; Tanaka, T. Uniaxial-isotropic metamaterials by three-dimensional split-ring resonators. *Adv. Opt. Mater.* **2015**, *3*, 44–48. [CrossRef]

34. Kuzel, P.; Kadlec, F.; Petzelt, J. Highly tunable SrTiO3/DyScO3 heterostructures for applications in the terahertz range. *Appl. Phys. Lett.* **2007**, *91*, 232911. [CrossRef]
35. LMartin, W.; Rappe, A.M. Thin-film ferroelectric materials and their applications. *Nat. Rev. Mater.* **2016**, *2*, 16087. [CrossRef]
36. Taira, T.; Saikawa, J.; Kobayashi, T.; Byer, R.L. Diode-pumped tunable Yb: YAG miniature lasers at room temperature: Modeling and experiment. *IEEE J. Sel. Top. Quantum Electron.* **1997**, *3*, 100–104. [CrossRef]
37. Lin, Z.; Wang, F.; Wang, M.; Zhang, L.; Feng, S.; Gao, G.; Wang, S.; Yu, C.; Hu, L. Maintaining broadband gain in a Nd^{3+}/Yb^{3+} co-doped silica fiber amplifier via dual-laser pumping. *Opt. Lett.* **2018**, *43*, 3361–3364. [CrossRef] [PubMed]
38. Manjappa, M.; Pitchappa, P.; Singh, N.; Wang, N.; Zheludev, N.; Lee, C.; Singh, R. Reconfigurable MEMS Fano metasurfaces with multiple-input-output states for logic operations at terahertz MEMS metamaterial. *Adv. Opt. Mater.* **2018**, *6*, 1800141. [CrossRef]
39. Cong, L.; Pitchappa, P.; Wu, Y.; Ke, L.; Lee, C.; Singh, N.; Yang, H.; Singh, R. Active multifunctional microelectromechanical system metadevices: Applications in polarization control, wavefront deflection and holograms. *Adv. Opt. Mater.* **2017**, *5*, 201600716. [CrossRef]
40. Pitchappa, P.; Manjappa, M.; Krishnamoorthy, H.N.S.; Chang, Y.; Lee, C.; Singh, R. Bidirectional reconfiguration and thermal tuning of microcantilever metamaterial device operating from 77 K to 400 K. *Appl. Phys. Lett.* **2017**, *111*, 261101. [CrossRef]
41. Davis, B.L.; Hussein, M.I. Nanophotonic metamaterial: Thermal conductivity reduction by local resonance. *Phys. Rev. Lett.* **2014**, *112*, 055505. [CrossRef]
42. Chen, C.; Pan, C.; Hsieh, C.F.; Lin, Y.; Pan, R. Liquid-crystal-based terahertz tunable Lyot filter. *Appl. Phys. Lett.* **2006**, *88*, 101107. [CrossRef]
43. Han, J.G.; Lakhtakia, A. Semiconductor split-ring resonators for thermally tunable terahertz metamaterials. *J. Mon. Opt.* **2009**, *56*, 554–557. [CrossRef]
44. Wen, Y.; Chen, K.; Lin, Y.-S. Terahertz metamaterial resonator with tunable Fano-resonance characteristic. *Results Phys.* **2021**, *23*, 104049. [CrossRef]
45. Xu, R.; Xu, X.; Yang, B.-R.; Gui, X.; Qin, Z.; Lin, Y.-S. Actively Logical Modulation of MEMS-Based Terahertz Metamaterial. *Photonics. Res.* **2021**, *9*, 1409–1415. [CrossRef]
46. Zhang, Y.; Lin, P.; Lin, Y.-S. Tunable Split-Disk Metamaterial Absorber for Sensing Application. *Nanomaterials* **2021**, *11*, 598. [CrossRef]
47. Wen, Y.; Liang, Z.; Lin, Y.-S. Tunable Perfect Meta-Absorber with High-Sensitive Polarization Characteristic. *Adv. Photon. Res.* **2021**, *2*, 2000027. [CrossRef]
48. Xu, T.; Xu, R.; Lin, Y.-S. Tunable Terahertz Metamaterial Using Electrostatically Electric Split-Ring Resonator. *Results Phys.* **2020**, *19*, 103638. [CrossRef]
49. Haynes, W.M. (Ed.) *CRC Handbook of Chemistry and Physics: A Ready-Reference Book of Chemical and Physical Data*, 97th ed.; CRC Press: Boca Raton, FL, USA, 2016.
50. Palik, E.D. *Handbook of Optical Constants of Solids*; Academic Press: San Diego, CA, USA, 1998.
51. Yahiaoui, R.; Tan, S.; Cong, L.; Singh, R.; Yan, F.; Zhang, W. Multispectral terahertz sensing with highly flexible ultrathin metamaterial absorber. *J. Appl. Phys.* **2015**, *118*, 083103. [CrossRef]

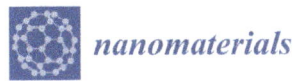

Article

Terahertz Metamaterial with Multiple Resonances for Biosensing Application

Huiliang Ou, Fangyuan Lu, Zefeng Xu and Yu-Sheng Lin *

State Key Laboratory of Optoelectronic Materials and Technologies, School of Electronics and Information Technology, Sun Yat-Sen University, Guangzhou 510275, China; ouhliang@mail2.sysu.edu.cn (H.O.); lufy@mail2.sysu.edu.cn (F.L.); xuzf6@mail2.sysu.edu.cn (Z.X.)
* Correspondence: linyoush@mail.sysu.edu.cn

Received: 7 May 2020; Accepted: 27 May 2020; Published: 29 May 2020

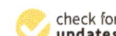

Abstract: A sickle-shaped metamaterial (SSM) based biochemical sensor with multiple resonances was investigated in the terahertz frequency range. The electromagnetic responses of SSM were found to be four resonances, namely dipolar, quadrupolar, octupolar and hexadecapolar plasmon resonances. They were generated from the interactions between SSM and perpendicularly incident terahertz waves. The sensing performances of SSM-based biochemical sensors were evaluated by changing ambient environments and analyte varieties. The highest values of sensitivity and figure of merit (FOM) for SSM covered with analyte thin-films were 471 GHz/RIU (refraction index unit) and 94 RIU^{-1}, respectively. In order to further investigate the biosensing ability of the proposed SSM device, dielectric hemispheres and microfluidic chips were adopted to imitate dry and hydrous biological specimens, respectively. The results show that the sensing abilities of SSM-based biochemical sensors could be enhanced by increasing either the number of hemispheres or the channel width of the microfluidic chip. The highest sensitivity was 405 GHz/RIU for SSM integrated with microfluidic chips. Finally, three more realistic models were simulated to imitate real sensing situations, and the corresponding highest sensitivity was 502 GHz/RIU. The proposed SSM device paves the way to possible uses in biochemical sensing applications.

Keywords: metamaterial; multiple resonances; biochemical sensing; environment sensor

1. Introduction

Recently, terahertz spectroscopy has attracted great interest due to its unique characteristics and availability in massively promising applications [1–3]. It has many photoelectric characteristics, such as low photon energy but high penetration, as well as non-contact and label-free inspection, which enable terahertz spectroscopy technology to detect chemicals and biomolecules [4,5]. In addition, terahertz waves are consistent with the inherent frequency of some important biomarkers, such as nucleic acid and specific proteins, which make terahertz biochemical sensors possible [6–8]. However, the optical properties of natural materials are inherent and cannot be changed. Moreover, terahertz waves' transmission is high for common plastics and fibers, and their reflectivity is also high for most metal materials. These optical properties represent a bottleneck for the interaction between natural materials and terahertz waves [9]. Metamaterial is a composite material that possesses unique electromagnetic properties realized by the configuration of specific structures. Near-field electromagnetic energy can interact and then be enhanced within the metamaterial. The combination of terahertz waves and metamaterial means that the incident electromagnetic wave can be controlled and manipulated.

The configuration of a metamaterial is a kind of synthetic subwavelength array structure which features negative permittivity, permeability, perfect absorption and superlens capability [10,11]. Metamaterial can be designed to possess single, dual, triple and multiple resonances by tailoring diversified metamaterial patterns and structures [12–14]. Among these plasmonic resonances, the frequency shift of higher-order plasmonic resonances with high quality factors (Q-factor) is ultrasensitive to the geometrical shapes and the local dielectric environment [15,16]. Therefore, plasmonic metamaterial-based sensors are usually compact, portable and cost-effective, possessing great potential for detecting different kinds of chemicals as well as biomolecules in trace amounts [17–19]. The utilization of plasmonic metamaterial-based sensors with high efficiency and high Q-factors is the essential reason for developing an ultrahigh-sensitivity biosensor.

In this study, a plasmonic metamaterial-based biochemical sensor with multiple resonances and high sensitivity is presented in the terahertz frequency range. The proposed plasmonic metamaterial is composed of an array of a pair of centrosymmetric sickle-shaped metamaterials (SSM). The ambient environments and analyte varieties were changed to investigate the sensitivity of SSM-based biochemical sensors. The higher-order plasmonic resonance was accompanied by a larger red-shifting of the resonance. The highest sensitivity was 471 GHz/RIU (refraction index unit) for the hexadecapolar plasmonic mode of SSM. The corresponding figure of merit (FOM) was 94 RIU^{-1}. We further investigated the influences of dielectric hemispheres and microfluidic chips to imitate the dry and hydrous biological specimens. The results show that the red-shifting of the resonance could be increased by raising the number of hemispheres and the channel width of the microfluidic chip. The relationships between resonance shifting, hemisphere quantity and the channel width of the microfluidic chip are quite linear. The proposed SSM device provides an effective approach to detecting and analyzing the chemicals and biomolecules.

2. Designs and Methods

Figure 1a shows a schematic drawing of the periodic SSM structure. The incident terahertz wave propagates perpendicularly to the SSM surface along the z-axis. A schematic diagram of an SSM unit cell is illustrated in Figure 1b, which includes the geometrical denotations. The SSM unit cell is composed of a pair of centrosymmetric Au split-ring resonators (SRRs) on a polydimethylsiloxane (PDMS) substrate. The permittivity of the Au material is described using the Drude model as expressed by [20–23]:

$$\varepsilon(\omega) = 1 - \frac{\omega_p^2}{\omega[(\omega + i\omega_c)]} \quad (1)$$

where $\omega_p = 1.37 \times 10^{16}$ Hz is the plasmon frequency and $\omega_c = 4.08 \times 10^{13}$ Hz is the scattering frequency for the Au material [20,24].

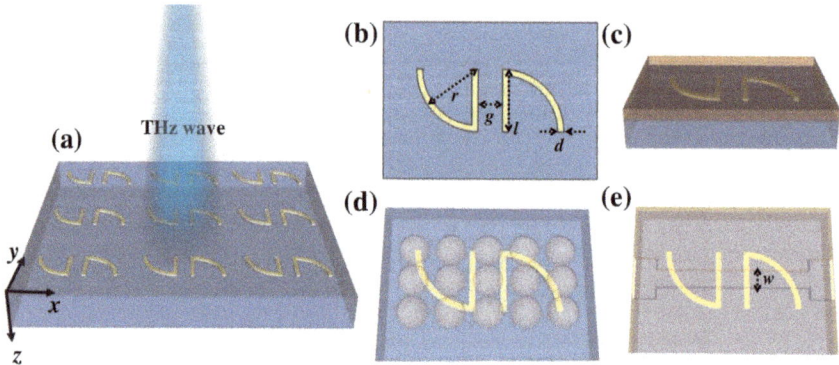

Figure 1. (a) Schematic drawing of the sickle-shaped metamaterial (SSM). (b) Geometrical denotations for the corresponding SSM unit cell. (c–e) Schematic drawings of SSM covered with (c) analyte thin-film, (d) dielectric hemispheres and (e) microfluidic channels.

Figure 1c shows the SSM device covered with an analyte thin-film serving as a chemical specimen. To further investigate the sensing of dry and aqueous biological specimens, dielectric hemispheres and microfluidic channels were integrated with the SSM device, as shown in Figure 1d,e. The full-field electromagnetic waves were simulated using the finite-difference time-domain (FDTD) method. In the numerical modeling, the periodic boundary conditions are adopted in both the x-axis and y-axis directions while the perfectly matched layer (PML) boundary condition is set in the z-axis direction. The incident polarized waves are defined as transverse electric (TE) and transverse magnetic (TM) modes when the electric (E) field of incident terahertz wave is along the x-axis and y-axis, respectively. To optimize the geometrical structures of the proposed SSM, the transmission spectra of SSM with different gaps between two SRRs (g) and thicknesses of Au layers (t) are shown in Figure 2. Figure 2a,b shows the transmission spectra of SSM with different t values in TE and TM modes. The transmission spectra are almost the same and there are no impacts in TE and TM modes. Therefore, the t value is defined as the average value of 200 nm in this study. Figure 2c,d shows the transmission spectra of SSM with different g values in TE and TM modes. The resonant intensities are almost the same and there is a little shift on the resonant frequencies. Since the variations of resonant frequencies have no significant influence on the sensing performance of SSM, the gap distance between SRRs is defined as 4 μm in this study. Other geometrical parameters are defined as follows: arc radius, r = 20 μm; width of Au lines, d = 2 μm; length of metallic bar, l = 20 μm (Figure 1b). The SSM period is 60 × 60 μm^2.

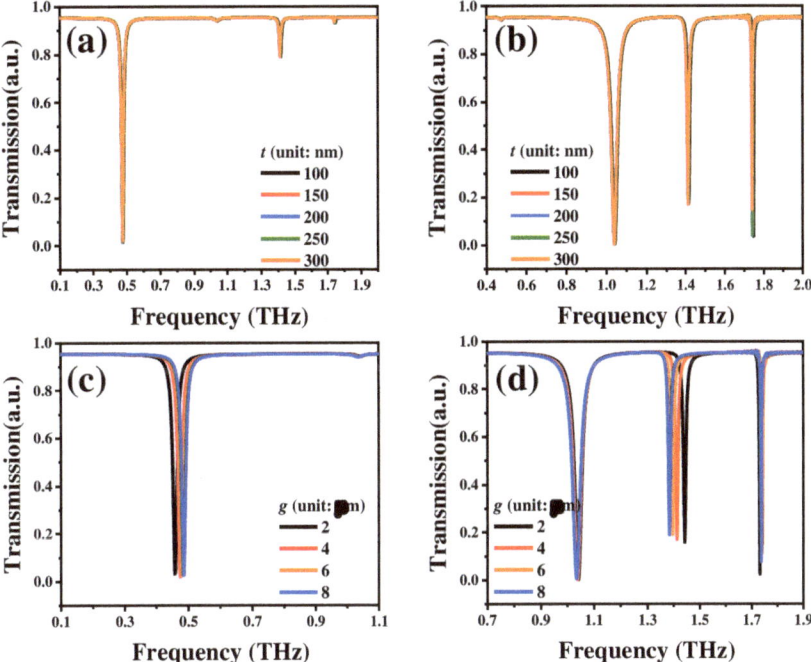

Figure 2. Transmission spectra of SSM with different t values in (**a**) transverse electric (TE)) and (**b**) transverse magnetic (TM) modes. Transmission spectra of SSM with different g values in (**c**) TE and (**d**) TM modes.

3. Results and Discussion

Figure 3a shows SSM transmission spectra in TE and TM modes under the condition of an environmental refraction index of 1.0. The geometrical parameters are kept constant at r = 20 μm,

$d = 2$ μm, $l = 20$ μm, $g = 4$ μm and $t = 200$ nm. Here, the environmental refraction index is denoted as n_b. A single resonance is at the lower frequency of 0.51 THz for the incident TE-polarized light, as the red curve shows in Figure 3a, while there are three resonances at the higher frequencies of 1.04, 1.44 and 1.73 THz for the incident TM-polarized light, as the blue curve shows in Figure 3a. The spectrum shape of the resonance is narrower at higher resonant frequencies than at lower resonant frequencies. This is one of the prominent characteristics of multipolar plasmon modes. In addition, the higher-order plasmon mode exhibits higher sensitivity in refraction-index sensing applications. The electromagnetic-field distributions of SSM at corresponding resonant frequencies are displayed to better understand the multipolar plasmon modes. The E- and H-fields of four resonances in the sorting orders are shown in Figure 3b–i. In Figure 3b, in terms of a single SRR, the E-field energy is mainly distributed on two sides, implying that this resonance is generated from the electric dipolar mode. Actually, the order of plasmon modes (o) satisfies the equation $o = n - 1$, where n is the number of notes in an open SRR [12]. For instance, the n and o values in Figure 3b are 2 and 1, respectively, and so the resonance mode at 0.51 THz is the fundamental plasmon resonance mode, i.e., the dipolar plasmon mode (D mode). Analogously, the orders of plasmon modes in Figure 3d, 3e and 3f are 2, 3 and 4, respectively. This indicates that the resonance modes at 1.04, 1.44 and 1.73 THz are quadrupolar (Q), octupolar (O) and hexadecapolar (H) plasmon-resonance modes, respectively. The phenomena of different plasmon modes excited by different polarized waves could be explained in terms of structural asymmetry and phases of internal fields. The gap in a split ring leads to polarization anisotropy and allows both odd and even plasmon modes to be excited. When the symmetrical structure is broken, that can be stimulated and then generate higher-order plasmon modes, such as Q and O modes [12,25,26]. The incident TE-polarized wave results in internal fields with opposite phases on both sides of the SRR. Therefore, the E-field energy is coupled with the SRR, generating the fundamental plasmon resonance, which is the dipolar mode, as the red curve shows in Figure 3a. When the incident polarized wave is perpendicular to the split gap, i.e., the TM mode, the confined electromagnetic fields are in same phases on both sides of the SRR. The even-order plasmon modes, such as Q and H modes, are thus generated, as the blue curve shows in Figure 3a. The O mode is generated from the electromagnetic wave excited in TM mode due to the mirror symmetrical structure being broken.

The strong localized E- and H-fields emerged on the designed SSM surface, which indicated that a sharp resonance with a high Q-factor will be generated. In order to utilize the above-mentioned merits of multiple resonances in biosensing applications, we further compared and analyzed the changes of the surrounding environments and analyte varieties and then covered the SSM surface with different dielectric hemispheres and microfluidic chips to investigate its influence on sensing performance. The environmental refraction index (n_b) was changed from 1.0 to 1.7 to verify the sensing ability of SSM. The transmission spectra of SSM with different n_b values in TM mode are shown in Figure 4a. There are three resonances at 1.04, 1.44 and 1.73 THz for the initial condition of $n_b = 1.0$. By increasing the n_b value, the resonances are apparently red-shifted and the resonant intensities kept stable. Figure 4b plots the relationships between frequency shifts and n_b values. The resonant frequencies are red-shifted linearly by increasing n_b values. The shifting range of H mode is the largest compared to that of Q and O modes. The sensitivity (S) of an SSM is defined as the derivative of the frequency shift with respect to the refraction index, i.e., the slopes of the dashed lines shown in Figure 4b. The calculated S values of Q, O and H modes were 286, 390 and 460 GHz/RIU, respectively. Furthermore, when the order of the plasmon mode increases, the resonance becomes sharper and the spectrum width is narrower. Q-factor is defined as the ratio of resonant frequency to the full width at half maximum (FWHM) transmission intensity, which is used to describe the quality of each resonant frequency. In Figure 4c, Q-factors of Q, O and H modes are quite stable and insensitive to n_b values. The average Q-factors are 33, 124 and 342 for Q, O and H modes, respectively. For biosensing performance, FOM is an important factor that determines the sensing abilities in the biochemical and biomolecule applications. FOM is defined by $S/FWMH$. The average FOM values of Q, O and H modes are 10, 37 and 100 RIU^{-1}, respectively, as plotted in Figure 4d. The sensing ability of SSM could be enhanced by increasing the order of plasmon modes.

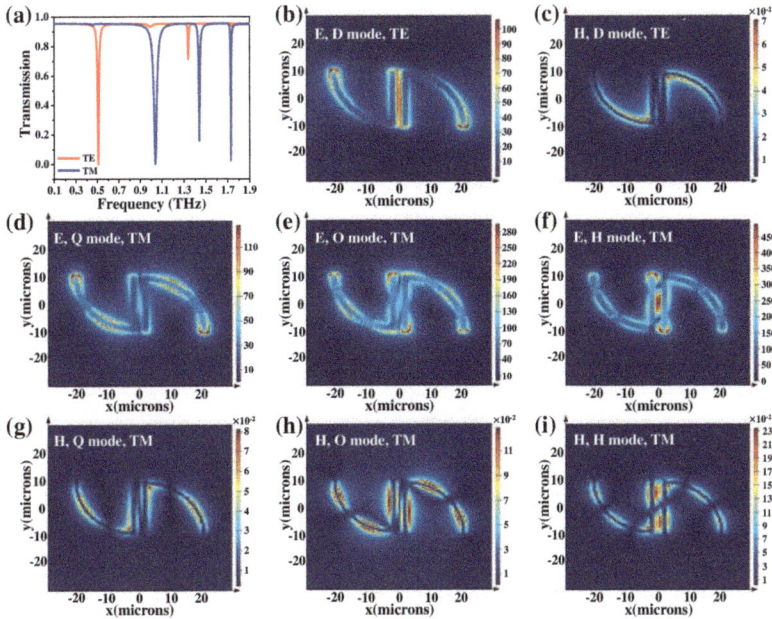

Figure 3. Transmission spectra of SSM and corresponding E- and H-field distributions. (**a**) Transmission spectra of SSM in TE and TM modes under the condition of $n_b = 1.0$. (**b**) E-field and (**c**) H-field distributions of SSM monitored in resonant dipolar mode (D mode) under the incident TE-polarized wave. (**d**–**f**) E-field and (**g**–**i**) H-field distributions of SSM monitored at resonant quadrupolar mode (Q mode), octupolar mode (O mode) and hexadecapolar mode (H mode) under the incident TM-polarized wave.

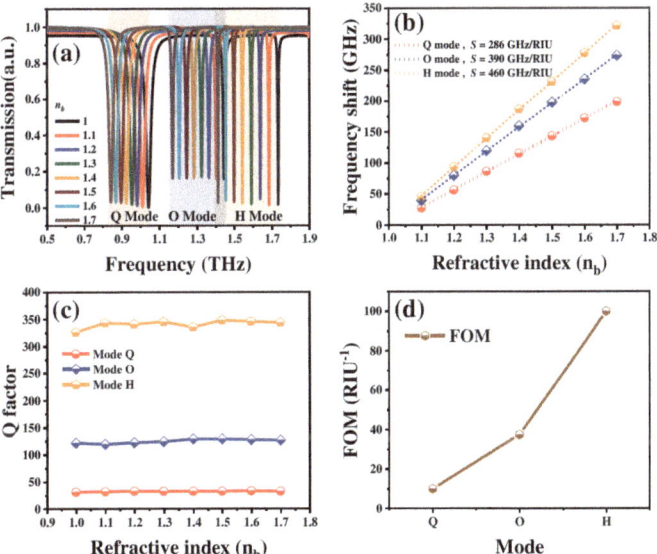

Figure 4. (**a**) Transmission spectra of SSM with different n_b values. (**b**) Frequency shifts and (**c**) Q-factors plotted against the n_b values. (**d**) The average figure of merit (FOM) values of Q, O and H modes.

We also investigated the effect of SSM covered with an analyte thin-film to compare the sensing ability of SSM. The refraction index of analyte thin-film is denoted as n_a. The thickness of analyte thin-film is 10 µm, as shown in Figure 1c. The transmission spectra of SSM with different n_a values from 1.0 to 1.35 are shown in Figure 5a. There are three resonances red-shifted by increasing n_a values. To express the red-shifts of three plasmon modes explicitly, the relationships of frequency shifts and n_a values are summarized in Figure 5b. The relationships are quite linear. The frequency-shift tendency reveals that the sensitivity of H mode (471 GHz/RIU) is higher than that of O mode (391 GHz/RIU) and of Q mode (281 GHz/RIU). To further obtain the quantitative descriptions for the sensing performances, Q-factors and FOM values of plasmon modes were calculated, as shown in Figure 5c,d, respectively. The average Q-factors of Q, O and H modes were 31, 112 and 328, respectively, while the average FOM values of Q, O and H modes were 9 RIU, 45 and 94 RIU^{-1}, respectively. The frequency-shift mechanism derived from the variation of n_a values can be explained by the perturbation theory [5,9,27,28].

$$\frac{\Delta\omega}{\omega_0} = \frac{\int_{\Delta V}(\mu|\overline{H}_0|_2 - \varepsilon|\overline{E}_0|_2)\mathrm{d}v}{\int_{v_0}(\varepsilon|\overline{E}_0|_2 + \mu|\overline{H}_0|_2)\mathrm{d}v} \quad (2)$$

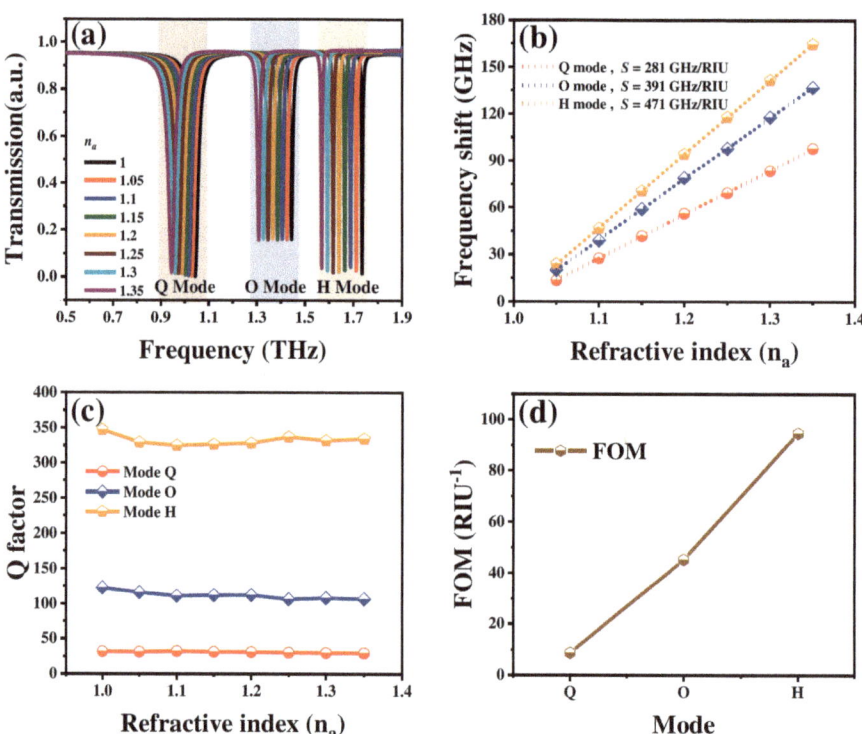

Figure 5. (a) Transmission spectra of SSM covered with different analyte thin-films. (b) Frequency shifts and (c) Q-factors plotted against the n_a values. (d) The average FOM values of Q, O and H modes. The dielectric hemispheres were introduced to imitate the detection of cells, such as the monitoring of cell apoptosis, as shown in Figure 1d. The refraction index of dielectric hemispheres (n_c) was investigated to study the electromagnetic behaviors of SSM for biosensing applications.

Here, perturbation means the variation of n_b values. E_0 and H_0 represent the unperturbed E-field and H-field, respectively. $\Delta\varepsilon$ ($\Delta\varepsilon = \varepsilon - \varepsilon_0$) and $\Delta\mu$ ($\Delta\mu = \mu - \mu_0$) are the changes to the dielectric constant and permeability after perturbation, respectively. $\Delta\omega$ ($\Delta\omega = \omega - \omega_0$) is the change to the resonant angular frequency and v_0 is the effective integral volume. It should be noted that Equation (2) is based on shape perturbations in terms of SSM. The perturbation is n_b, with no v_0. In addition, the effect of permeability on frequency shifts is negligible since the proposed SSM is non-magnetic. Therefore, it can be expressed by:

$$\frac{\Delta\omega}{\omega_0} = \frac{-\int_{v_0} \Delta\varepsilon |\overline{E}_0|^2 dv}{\int_{v_0} (\varepsilon|\overline{E}_0|_2 + \mu|\overline{H}_0|_2) dv} \qquad (3)$$

It can be seen that the $\Delta\varepsilon$ value decreases by increasing the n_b value according to $n_b = \sqrt{\mu_r \varepsilon_r}$. Consequently, the $\Delta\omega$ value decreases and the resonant frequency is then red-shifted.

Figure 6a shows the transmission spectra of SSM covered with different hemispheres under the condition of a hemisphere quantity of 15. The resonances are red-shifted by increasing n_c values from 1.0 to 1.6. This indicates that the proposed SSM device has the ability to sense biological cells with different refraction indices. The relationships of n_c values and frequency shifts are summarized in Figure 6b. SSM exhibits an effective frequency shift by increasing the hemisphere number or plasmon mode. For example, when the hemisphere number is fixed at 10, as the blue plane shows in Figure 6b, the resonances are red-shifted with a slope of 262 for H mode. This is larger than that of O mode (slope = 174) and of Q mode (slope = 119). Moreover, when the n_c value is kept constant, the frequency shifts become larger by increasing the hemisphere number. The proposed SSM is useful for the detection of cell proliferation or cell apoptosis. When the plasmon mode is determined, the resonances are red-shifted with a slope of 359 for a hemisphere number of 15 in H mode. This is larger than that for a hemisphere number of 10 (slope = 262) and a hemisphere number of 5 (slope = 97) in H mode. The above-mentioned results indicate that the biosensing performance of SSM could be enhanced by either utilizing higher plasmon-oscillation modes or increasing the concentration of biomolecules.

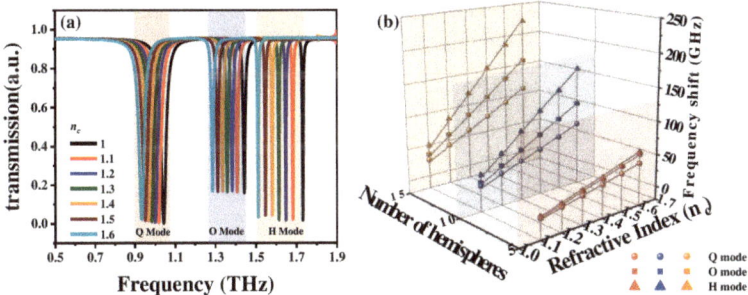

Figure 6. (**a**) Transmission spectra of SSM covered with different hemispheres under the condition of a hemisphere quantity of 15. (**b**) Summaries of the relationships of frequency shifts and n_c values and hemisphere quantities.

We further investigated the sensing performance of SSM integrated with a microfluidic chip. This has great potential for sensing biosamples, owing to the fact that most biological specimens are dissolved in aqueous environments. Furthermore, the requirement for an injected analyte sample is micro-/nanoliters. This minute amount of analyte sample can significantly prevent the terahertz absorption of the water and thus improve the sensing capacity of SSM. The thickness and width of the microfluidic channel are 20 μm and w, as shown in Figure 1e. The microfluidic channel is superimposed on the split gaps of SSM, i.e., the region with strongest E-field energy. Therefore, the resonances of SSM could be tuned by injecting different chemical solutions into the microfluidic channel. Here, the refraction index for injecting chemical solutions into the microfluidic channel is denoted as n_s.

Figure 7a shows the transmission spectra of SSM with different n_s values from 1.0 to 1.6, keeping w constant at 10 μm. SSM exhibits three resonances with consistently resonant intensities under the variation of n_s values. These three resonances are red-shifted by increasing n_s values for Q, O and H modes. The relationships between frequency shifts, n_s values and w values are summarized in Figure 7b. The relationships are kept linear between frequency shifts and n_s values by keeping the channel width constant. The resonances are red-shifted by increasing the plasmon orders. When a resonant plasmon mode is determined, the frequency shifts can be enhanced by enlarging the microfluidic channel width. Therefore, the highest sensitivity of an SSM integrated with microfluidic chip emerged in H mode when the channel width was 20 μm; this was 405 GHz/RIU. These results imply that the SSM device is ultrasensitive to the variation of the surrounding environment and thus is a potential platform for biosensing biological specimens.

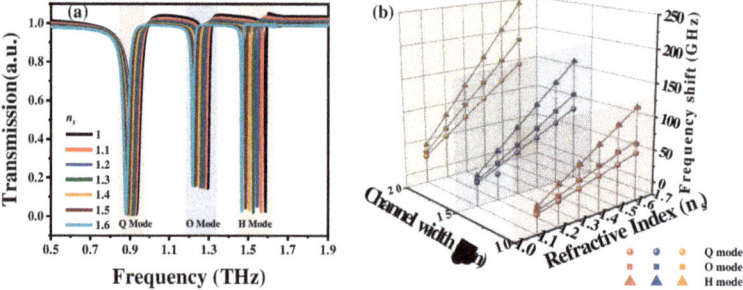

Figure 7. (**a**) Transmission spectra of SSM integrated with a microfluidic chip. The chemical solutions with different refraction indexes (n_s) are injected into the microfluidic channel with a channel width of 10 μm. (**b**) Summaries of relationships between frequency shifts, n_s values and channel widths.

In consideration of the realistic materials, including rough PDMS, crude analyte thin-films and irregular biological cells, three more realistic models were simulated to imitate real situations. The schematics of the top views of SSM on a rough PDMS substrate, covered with crude analyte thin-film and covered with random ellipse particles are shown in Figure 8a–c. The roughness of the PDMS surface and the analyte thin-film was introduced by texturing surfaces, with the maximum texturing depth determined to be 200 nm. The random ellipse particles were introduced by determining three ellipse radii haphazardly in the range of 3 to 5 μm. Figure 8d shows the transmission spectra of SSM on rough PDMS substrates with increasing n_b values. The resonances are red-shifted significantly compared to those results in Figure 4a. This implies that the sensing capacity of SSM can be enhanced by texturing the substrate surface. The relationships between frequency shifts and n_b values are summarized in Figure 8g. The sensitivities are 302 GHz/RIU for Q mode, 414 GHz/RIU for O mode and 502 GHz/RIU for H mode, which are greater than those results in Figure 4b (286, 390 and 460 GHz/RIU for Q, O H modes, respectively). These enhancements are due to the additional space below the metallic SRRs after texturing the PDMS surface. Figure 8e shows the transmission spectra of SSM covered with crude analyte thin-films with different n_c values. The sensitivities of Q, O and H modes are 26, 36 and 49 GHz/RIU, respectively, which are lower than those in Figure 5a. Figure 8f shows the transmission spectra of SSM covered with random ellipse particles with different n_c values. The sensitivities are 103, 158 and 258 GHz/RIU for Q, O and H modes, respectively. These values are lower than those in Figure 6b. As mentioned above, the sensitivity could be improved by increasing the hemisphere number and channel width of the microfluidic chip. This proves that the results of the lower sensitivities in Figure 8h,i, caused by the rough analyte thin-film and the deformation of ellipse particles owing to the coupling effects, are minor for SSM covered with a crude analyte thin-film and random ellipse particles.

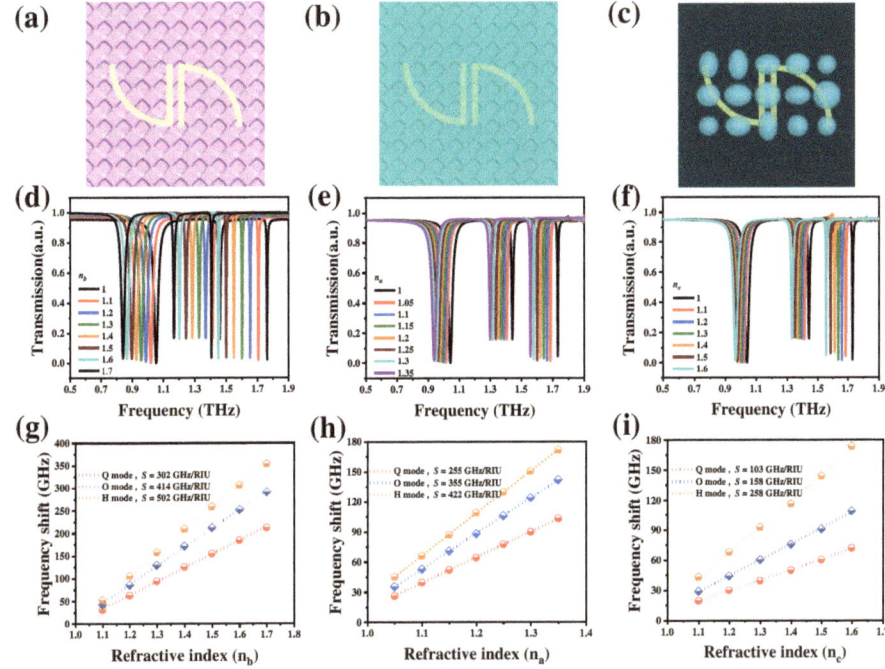

Figure 8. Schematics of top views of SSM (**a**) on a rough polydimethylsiloxane (PDMS) substrate, (**b**) covered with a crude analyte thin-film and (**c**) covered with random ellipse particles. (**d–f**) Transmission spectra of SSM (**d**) on rough PDMS substrate with different n_b values, (**e**) covered with different crude analyte thin-films and (**f**) covered with different random ellipse particles. (**g–i**) The summaries of the relationships between the frequency shifts and refraction indexes of (**d–f**).

4. Conclusions

In conclusion, an SSM-based biochemical sensor composed of centrosymmetric Au SRRs on a PDMS substrate was proposed and investigated in the terahertz wavelength. By changing different surrounding dielectric environments, the sensing performance of the proposed biosensor was verified. The results show that the increments of environmental refraction indexes (n_b, n_a, n_c and n_s) lead to the apparent red-shifts of resonances in the terahertz frequency range. Furthermore, the higher plasmon mode exhibits larger frequency shifts and greater sensitivity in biosensing applications. The dielectric hemispheres and microfluidic channels are further integrated into the proposed SSM device to verify the biosensing abilities of SSM. This indicates that the increments of hemisphere concentration or microfluidic channel width are beneficial for improving the sensing performance of an SSM-based biosensor. The highest sensitivity was 471 GHz/RIU. Finally, we propose three more realistic models to more reasonably mimic a real sensing situation, and the corresponding highest sensitivity was 502 GHz/RIU. This proposed SSM is quite suitable for use in biochemical and biomedical sensing applications.

Author Contributions: Conceptualization, H.O. and Y.-S.L.; methodology, H.O., F.L., Z.X. and Y.-S.L.; formal analysis, H.O.; investigation, H.O., F.L.; data curation, H.O., F.L., Z.X.; writing—original draft preparation, H.O.; writing—review and editing, Y.-S.L.; visualization, Y.-S.L.; supervision, Y.-S.L.; funding acquisition, Y.-S.L. All authors have read and agreed to the published version of the manuscript.

Funding: This research was funded by National Key Research and Development Program of China (2019YFA0705000).

Acknowledgments: The authors acknowledge the State Key Laboratory of Optoelectronic Materials and Technologies of Sun Yat-Sen University, for the use of experimental equipment.

Conflicts of Interest: The authors declare no conflict of interest.

References

1. Liu, P.; Liang, Z.; Lin, Z.; Xu, Z.; Xu, R.; Yao, D.; Lin, Y.-S. Actively tunable terahertz chain-link metamaterial with bidirectional polarization-dependent characteristic. *Sci. Rep.* **2019**, *9*, 9917. [CrossRef]
2. Xu, Z.; Lin, Z.; Cheng, S.; Lin, Y.-S. Reconfigurable and tunable terahertz wrench-shape metamaterial performing programmable characteristic. *Opt. Lett.* **2019**, *44*, 3944–3947. [CrossRef] [PubMed]
3. Xu, Z.; Lin, Y.-S. A Stretchable Terahertz Parabolic-Shaped Metamaterial. *Adv. Opt. Mater.* **2019**, *7*, 1900379. [CrossRef]
4. Salim, A.; Lim, S. Review of Recent Metamaterial Microfluidic Sensors. *Sensors* **2018**, *18*, 232. [CrossRef]
5. Zhang, Z.; Ding, H.; Yan, X.; Liang, L.; Wei, D.; Wang, M.; Yang, Q.; Yao, J. Sensitive detection of cancer cell apoptosis based on the non-bianisotropic metamaterials biosensors in terahertz frequency. *Opt. Mater. Express* **2018**, *8*, 659–667. [CrossRef]
6. Geng, Z.; Zhang, X.; Fan, Z.; Lv, X.; Chen, H. A Route to Terahertz Metamaterial Biosensor Integrated with Microfluidics for Liver Cancer Biomarker Testing in Early Stage. *Sci. Rep.* **2017**, *7*, 16378. [CrossRef]
7. Lan, F.; Luo, F.; Mazumder, P.; Yang, Z.; Meng, L.; Bao, Z.; Zhou, J.; Zhang, Y.; Liang, S.; Shi, Z.; et al. Dual-band refractometric terahertz biosensing with intense wave-matter-overlap microfluidic channel. *Biomed. Opt. Express* **2019**, *10*, 3789–3799. [CrossRef]
8. Lee, S.-H.; Choe, J.-H.; Kim, C.; Bae, S.; Kim, J.-S.; Park, Q.-H.; Seo, M. Graphene assisted terahertz metamaterials for sensitive bio-sensing. *Sens. Actuators B Chem.* **2020**, *310*, 127841. [CrossRef]
9. Yang, M.; Zhang, Z.; Liang, L.; Yan, X.; Wei, D.; Song, X.; Zhang, H.; Lu, Y.; Wang, M.; Yao, J. Sensitive detection of the concentrations for normal epithelial cells based on Fano resonance metamaterial biosensors in terahertz range. *Appl. Opt.* **2019**, *58*, 6268–6273. [CrossRef]
10. Lin, Z.; Xu, Z.; Liu, P.; Liang, Z.; Lin, Y.-S. Polarization-sensitive terahertz resonator using asymmetrical F-shaped metamaterial. *Opt. Laser Technol.* **2020**, *121*, 105826. [CrossRef]
11. Lu, F.; Ou, H.; Liao, Y.; Zhu, F.; Lin, Y.-S. Actively switchable terahertz metamaterial. *Results Phys.* **2019**, *15*, 102756. [CrossRef]
12. Sheridan, A.K.; Clark, A.; Glidle, A.; Cooper, J.M.; Cumming, D.R.S. Multiple plasmon resonances from gold nanostructures. *Appl. Phys. Lett.* **2007**, *90*, 143105. [CrossRef]
13. Yang, M.; Liang, L.; Zhang, Z.; Xin, Y.; Wei, D.; Song, X.; Zhang, H.; Lu, Y.; Wang, M.; Zhang, M.; et al. Electromagnetically induced transparency-like metamaterials for detection of lung cancer cells. *Opt. Express* **2019**, *27*, 19520–19529. [CrossRef] [PubMed]
14. Zhao, L.; Liu, H.; He, Z.; Dong, S. Theoretical design of twelve-band infrared metamaterial perfect absorber by combining the dipole, quadrupole, and octopole plasmon resonance modes of four different ring-strip resonators. *Opt. Express* **2018**, *26*, 12838–12851. [CrossRef] [PubMed]
15. Fu, Y.H.; Zhang, J.B.; Yu, Y.F.; Luk'Yanchuk, B. Generating and Manipulating Higher Order Fano Resonances in Dual-Disk Ring Plasmonic Nanostructures. *ACS Nano* **2012**, *6*, 5130–5137. [CrossRef]
16. Guo, X.; Hu, H.; Zhu, X.; Yang, X.; Dai, Q. Higher order Fano graphene metamaterials for nanoscale optical sensing. *Nanoscale* **2017**, *9*, 14998–15004. [CrossRef]
17. Tang, W.; Wang, L.; Chen, X.; Liu, C.; Yu, A.; Lu, W. Dynamic Metamaterial based on the Graphene Split Ring High-Q Fano-resonnator for Sensing Applications. *Nanoscale* **2016**, *8*, 15196–15204. [CrossRef]
18. Yan, X.; Zhang, Z.; Liang, L.; Yang, M.; Wei, D.; Song, X.; Zhang, H.; Lu, Y.; Liu, L.; Zhang, M.; et al. A multiple mode integrated biosensor based on higher order Fano metamaterials. *Nanoscale* **2020**, *12*, 1719–1727. [CrossRef]

19. Verellen, N.; Van Dorpe, P.; Huang, C.; Lodewijks, K.; VandenBosch, G.A.E.; Lagae, L.; Moshchalkov, V.V. Plasmon Line Shaping Using Nanocrosses for High Sensitivity Localized Surface Plasmon Resonance Sensing. *Nano Lett.* **2011**, *11*, 391–397. [CrossRef]
20. Zhang, J.; Fan, W.; Panoiu, N.C.; Malloy, K.J.; Brueck, S.R.J.; Osgood, R.M. Experimental Demonstration of Near-Infrared Negative-Index Metamaterials. *Phys. Rev. Lett.* **2005**, *95*, 137404. [CrossRef]
21. Johnson, P.B.; Christy, R.W. Optical Constants of the Noble Metals. *Phys. Rev. B* **1972**, *6*, 4370–4379. [CrossRef]
22. Sehmi, H.S.; Langbein, W.W.; Muljarov, E.A. Optimizing the Drude-Lorentz model for material permittivity: Method, program, and examples for gold, silver, and copper. *Phys. Rev. B* **2017**, *95*, 115444. [CrossRef]
23. Zhong, M.; Jiang, X.; Zhu, X.; Zhang, J.; Zhong, J. Design and fabrication of a single metal layer tunable metamaterial absorber in THz range. *Opt. Laser Technol.* **2020**, *125*, 106023. [CrossRef]
24. Liu, N.; Langguth, L.; Weiss, T.; Kästel, J.; Fleischhauer, M.; Pfau, T.; Giessen, H. Plasmonic analogue of electromagnetically induced transparency at the Drude damping limit. *Nat. Mater.* **2009**, *8*, 758–762. [CrossRef]
25. Zhang, Y.; Jia, T.; Xu, Z.Z. Fano resonances in disk–ring plasmonic nanostructure: Strong interaction between bright dipolar and dark multipolar mode. *Opt. Lett.* **2012**, *37*, 4919. [CrossRef]
26. Rockstuhl, C.; Lederer, F.; Etrich, C.; Zentgraf, T.; Kuhl, J.; Giessen, H. On the reinterpretation of resonances in split-ring-resonators at normal incidence. *Opt. Express* **2006**, *14*, 8827–8836. [CrossRef]
27. Zhang, C.; Liang, L.; Ding, L.; Jin, B.; Hou, Y.; Li, C.; Jiang, L.; Liu, W.; Hu, W.; Lu, Y.; et al. Label-free measurements on cell apoptosis using a terahertz metamaterial-based biosensor. *Appl. Phys. Lett.* **2016**, *108*, 241105. [CrossRef]
28. David, M. *Microwave Engineering*, 4th ed.; John Wiley & Sons, Inc.: Hoboken, NJ, USA, 2011; p. 309.

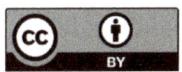

© 2020 by the authors. Licensee MDPI, Basel, Switzerland. This article is an open access article distributed under the terms and conditions of the Creative Commons Attribution (CC BY) license (http://creativecommons.org/licenses/by/4.0/).

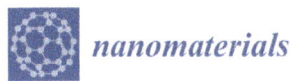

Review

High Potency of Organic and Inorganic Nanoparticles to Treat Cystic Echinococcosis: An Evidence-Based Review

Aishah E. Albalawi [1], Abdullah D. Alanazi [2], Parastoo Baharvand [3], Maryam Sepahvand [4] and Hossein Mahmoudvand [5,*]

1. Faculty of Science, University of Tabuk, Tabuk 47912, Saudi Arabia; ae.albalawii@ut.edu.sa
2. Department of Biological Science, Faculty of Science and Humanities, Shaqra University, P.O. Box 1040, Ad-Dawadimi 11911, Saudi Arabia; aalanazi@su.edu.sa
3. Department of Social Medicine, School of Medicine, Lorestan University of Medical Sciences, Khorramabad 6813833946, Iran; dr.baharvand@gmail.com
4. Student Research Committee, Lorestan University of Medical Sciences, Khorramabad 6813833946, Iran; msepahv@gmail.com
5. Razi Herbal Medicines Research Center, Lorestan University of Medical Sciences, Khorramabad 6813833946, Iran
* Correspondence: dmahmodvand@gmail.com

Received: 19 October 2020; Accepted: 14 December 2020; Published: 17 December 2020

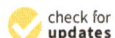

Abstract: Since there is no potential, effective vaccine available, treatment is the only controlling option against hydatid cyst or cystic echinococcosis (CE). This study was designed to systematically review the in vitro, in vivo, and ex vivo effects of nanoparticles against hydatid cyst. The study was carried out based on the 06- PRISMA guideline and registered in the CAMARADES-NC3Rs Preclinical Systematic Review and Meta-analysis Facility (SyRF) database. The search was performed in five English databases, including Scopus, PubMed, Web of Science, EMBASE, and Google Scholar without time limitation for publications around the world about the protoscolicdal effects of all the organic and inorganic nanoparticles without date limitation in order to identify all the published articles (in vitro, in vivo, and ex vivo). The searched words and terms were: "nanoparticles", "hydatid cyst", "protoscoleces", "cystic echinococcosis", "metal nanoparticles", "organic nanoparticles", "inorganic nanoparticles, "in vitro", ex vivo", "in vivo". Out of 925 papers, 29 papers including 15 in vitro (51.7%), 6 in vivo (20.7%), ex vivo 2 (6.9%), and 6 in vitro/in vivo (20.7%) up to 2020 met the inclusion criteria for discussion in this systematic review. The results demonstrated the most widely used nanoparticles in the studies were metal nanoparticles such as selenium, silver, gold, zinc, copper, iron nanoparticles (n = 8, 28.6%), and metal oxide nanoparticles such as zinc oxide, titanium dioxide, cerium oxide, zirconium dioxide, and silicon dioxide (n = 8, 28.6%), followed by polymeric nanoparticles such as chitosan and chitosan-based nanoparticles (n = 7, 25.0%). The results of this review showed the high efficacy of a wide range of organic and inorganic NPs against CE, indicating that nanoparticles could be considered as an alternative and complementary resource for CE treatment. The results demonstrated that the most widely used nanoparticles for hydatid cyst treatment were metal nanoparticles and metal oxide nanoparticles, followed by polymeric nanoparticles. We found that the most compatible drugs with nanoparticles were albendazole, followed by praziquantel and flubendazole, indicating a deeper understanding about the synergistic effects of nanoparticles and the present anti-parasitic drugs for treating hydatid cysts. The important point about using these nanoparticles is their toxicity; therefore, cytotoxicity as well as acute and chronic toxicities of these nanoparticles should be considered in particular. As a limitation, in the present study, although most of the studies have been performed in vitro, more studies are needed to confirm the effect of these nanoparticles as well as their exact mechanisms in the hydatid cyst treatment, especially in animal models and clinical settings.

Keywords: hydatid cyst; protoscoleces; nanomedicine; in vitro; in vivo; ex vivo

1. Background

Hydatid cyst or cystic echinococcosis (CE) is well-known as one of the most common universal parasitic infections, which infects a wide range of hosts such as humans, wild animals, and domestic livestock [1]. Therefore, CE can be considered as an important challenge both from medical and economic points of view [2]. In humans, hydatid cyst occurs through accidental infection with ingesting eggs of *Echinococcus granulosus* (dog tapeworm) expelled from the dog as the final host, followed by the growth of the larvae stage and transformation into cyst, predominantly in the liver (nearly 70%), and less frequently in the lungs, spleen, kidneys, and brain [3]. Considering the clinical symptoms of hydatid cyst, the onset of the disease shows no specific symptoms; but depending on the number, location, and size, the cysts have variable symptoms from mild to deadly [4].

Since there is no potential, effective vaccine available, treatment is the only controlling option against hydatid cyst diseases. Today, the therapeutic approaches for hydatid cyst treatment are medical treatment, surgical treatment, endoscopic interventional treatment, percutaneous methods (puncture, aspiration, injection, and re-aspiration (PAIR)), as well as the consequent minimally invasive techniques [5]. Therefore, in small and inactive cysts, the preferred treatment is chemotherapy with benzimidazole derivatives (mebendazole and albendazole); however, the first choice treatment for large and active cysts is surgery [6].

The results of recent studies have shown chemotherapy with benzimidazole derivatives is associated with some side-effects, i.e., hepatotoxicity, teratogenicity, methemoglobinemia, severe leucopenia, thrombocytopenia, and osteoporosis, indicating that caution should be exercised in using of these drugs [6]. By surgical treatment, since the rupture of cysts or leakage of their contents (protoscoleces) may cause re-infection, secondary infection, as well as anaphylaxis shock, surgeons use a number of chemical protoscolicidal agents such as hypertonic saline 20%, silver nitrate, and formalin to prevent these complications [4]. Hence, recent studies have demonstrated that the current protoscolicidal agents are not risk-free and can cause complications such as biliary fibrosis, hepatic necrosis, and cirrhosis [4,7]. Therefore, searching and discovering a new protoscolicidal agent are of top priority for physicians in this field.

Nanomedicine is considered as a relatively new field of science and technology that deals with nanometer-sized materials for medical purposes [8]. To date, nanomedicine has a variety of diagnostic and therapeutic applications in modern medicine, such as drug delivery, imaging, diagnosis, medical devices, vaccines, as well as antimicrobial therapy [9]. Considering applications of nanomedicine in treating microbial diseases, a wide range of studies have reported the antimicrobial effects of some inorganic nanoparticles (such as metal and metal oxide) and organic nanoparticles (peptide- and polymer-based nanoparticles such as cationic peptides, synthetic cationic polymers, chitosan, etc.) [10–12]. Considering the protoscolicidal activity of nanoparticles, although Shnawa et al. [13] reviewed the application of nanomedicine, especially green biosynthesis nanoparticles such as biogenic selenium, silver, gold, and chitosan nanoparticles, as new protoscolicidal alternative to treat hydatid cysts [13], in this study, we aim to systematically review the in vitro, in vivo, and ex vivo effects of a wide range of nanoparticles such as metal, carbon-based nanoparticles, lipid-based nanoparticles, polymeric nanoparticles, etc. against hydatid cyst.

2. Materials and Methods

2.1. Search Strategy

The current study was carried out based on 06- PRISMA guideline [14] and registered in the CAMARADES-NC3Rs Preclinical Systematic Review and Meta-analysis Facility (SyRF) database.

The search was performed in five English databases, including Scopus, PubMed, Web of Science, EMBASE, and Google Scholar without time limitation for publications worldwide on the protoscolicidal effects of organic and inorganic nanoparticles without date limitation in order to identify all the published articles (in vitro, in vivo, and ex vivo). Studies in any languages were entered in the search step if they had an English abstract. The words and terms were used as a syntax with specific tags of each database. The searched words and terms were: "protoscolicidal", "scolicidal", "nanoparticles", "hydatid cyst", "metal nanoparticles", "protoscoleces", "cystic echinococcosis", "in vitro", ex vivo", "in vivo", "scolex" etc. (Figure 1).

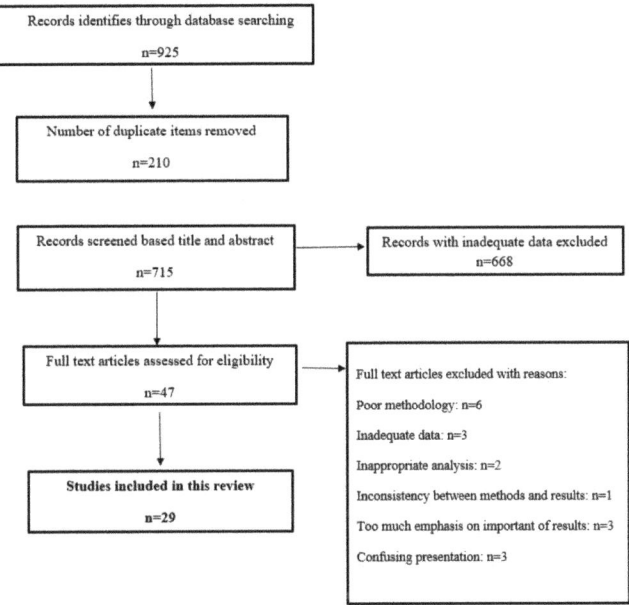

Figure 1. Flowchart describing the study design process.

2.2. Quality Assessment and Article Selection

Those studies were examined, in which the effects of nanoparticles against hydatid cyst were investigated. First, the studies were imported into EndNote X9 software (Thomson Reuters, New York, NY, USA) and duplicate studies were deleted. Afterwards, three independent authors examined the title and abstract of the studies and relevant works were included for further analysis. The same authors carefully read the studies and the eligible studies with adequate inclusion criteria were selected.

2.3. Exclusion Criteria

The studies with inadequate information, abstract submitted in congresses, full texts of which were not available, and failure to match methods with the incorrect interpretation of the results was excluded from the current study.

2.4. Inclusion Criteria

Inclusion criteria of this study were the articles evaluating the in vitro, ex vivo, and in vivo effects of various forms of nanoparticles containing drugs and other pharmaceutical formulations of organic and non-organic nanoparticles against hydatid cyst (Figure 1).

2.5. Data Extraction

Three independent authors extracted information from the selected articles and, if needed, the differences were resolved by the corresponding author. The extracted data included nanoparticle type, in combination or loaded with other drugs, type of study, animal model, concentration, time of use, reference, etc.

3. Results

Out of 925 papers, 29 papers including 15 in vitro (51.7%), 6 in vivo (20.7%), ex vivo 2 (6.9%), and 6 in vitro/in vivo (20.7%) up to 2020 met the inclusion criteria for discussion in this systematic review, the extracted data of which are presented in Tables 1–3. The most common type of nanoparticles were organic nanoparticles (15 studies, 51.7%) such as polymeric, lipid, etc., followed by non-organic nanoparticles such as metal and metal oxide nanoparticles (14 studies, 48.3%). The results demonstrated that the most widely used nanoparticles in the studies were metal nanoparticles such as selenium, silver, gold, zinc, copper, and iron nanoparticles (n = 8, 28.6%), metal oxide nanoparticles such as zinc oxide, titanium dioxide, cerium oxide, zirconium dioxide, and silicon dioxide (n = 8, 28.6%), followed by polymeric nanoparticles such as chitosan and chitosan based nanoparticles (n = 7, 25.0%). The findings also showed that, in the in vitro studies, the best exposure times were 60 min (n = 13, 46.4%), followed by 10 min (n = 4, 14.3%) and 120 min (n = 3, 10.7%). The results exhibited that the doses used in the in vitro studies were ranging from 0.0005 to 20 mg/kg, whereas in the in vivo studies, the doses ranged from 0.5 to 100 mg/kg.

Table 1. A list of in vitro studies on effects of nanoparticles against hydtid cysts.

Nanoparticles	Drug	Outcome		Ref
		Concentration of Drug (µg/mL)	Best Exposure Time	
Solid lipid nanoparticles (SLNs)	Albendazole Loaded SLN	250	Fifth day	[15]
		500	Fifth day	
		2	72 h	[16]
	Albendazole Sulfoxide Loaded SLN	2	72 h	[17]
		2.5		
		2	72 h	[16]
Lipid nanocapsules (LNCs)	Albendazole -LNCs	0.5	-	[18]
		1	-	
		1.5	7 day	
Nano lipid carriers (NLCs)	NLCs Loaded Ivermectin	50	-	[19]
		100	-	
		200	150 min	
		400	120 min	
		800	60 min	
Metal NPs	Selenium NPs	50	-	[20]
		125	-	
		250	20 min	
		500	10 min	
		50	-	[21]
		125	-	
		250	-	
		500	60 min	
	Silver NPs	500	-	[22]
		1000	-	
		2000	-	
		4000	60 min	
		25	-	[23]
		50	-	
		100	-	
		150	120 min	
		50	-	[21]
		125	-	
		250	60 min	
		500	-	
		250	-	[24]
		500	-	
		1000	60 min	

Table 1. Cont.

Nanoparticles	Drug		Outcome		Ref
			Concentration of Drug (μg/mL)	Best Exposure Time	
	Gold NPs		50	-	[25]
			100	-	
			200	-	
			300	120 min	
			250	-	[26]
			500	-	
			1000	-	
			2000	-	
			4000	60 min	
			250	-	[27]
			500	-	
			1000	60 min	
	Zinc NPs		250	10 min	[24]
			500	-	
			1000	-	
	Copper NPs		250	-	[24]
			500	60 min	
			1000	-	
	Iron NPs		250	-	[24]
			500	10 min	
			1000	-	
Metal oxide NPs	Zinc Oxide NPs		50,000	10 min	[28]
			10,000	-	
	Sea Urchin Gonad Extraction Combined with TiO2 NPs		1	-	[29]
			5	-	
			15	60 min	
	CeO2 NPs		1000	-	[30]
			5000	-	
			10,000	-	
			15,000	-	
			20,000	60 min	
	ZrO2		250	-	[31]
			500	-	
			1000	60 min	
			2000	60 min	
			4000	60 min	
Nonmetals oxide NPs	SiO2 NPs		250	-	[24]
			500	-	
			1000	60 min	
Nanopolymeric particles	Chitosan NPs	Curcumin	500	-	[32]
			1000	-	
			2000	-	
			4000	60 min	
		Praziquantel	1	-	[33]
			5	Tenth days	
			10	Tenth days	
		Albendazole	1	-	[33]
			5	Tenth days	
			10	Tenth days	
	Albendazole Sulfoxide Loaded PLGA-PEG NPs		50	-	[34]
			100	-	
			150	All The time	
			200	All The time	
	Flubendazole-Loaded mPEG-PCL NPs		1	-	[35]
			5	-	
			10	Fifteenth days	

Table 2. A list of in vivo studies on effects of nanoparticles against hydtid cysts.

Group		Drug	Animal	Drug Dose	Outcome Duration of Medication	Investigation Timeframe	Ref.
Nanopolymeric particles		Flubendazole-loaded mPEG-PCL NPs	BALB/c mice	5 mg/kg	1 month	8 months	[35]
	Chitosan NPs	Praziquantel	Male DBA/2 mice	25mg/kg	21 days	8 months	[33]
		Albendazole	Male DBA/2 Mice	25 mg/kg	21 days	8 months	[33]
		Albendazole sulfoxide (ABZ-SO)-loaded chitosan-PLGA nanoparticles	BALB/c mice	10 mg/kg	45 days	10 months	[36]
Metal oxide NPs		CeO2 NPs	Male BALB/c mice	50 mg/kg	1 month	2 months	[30]
		Sea Urchin Gonad Extraction Combined with Tio2 NPs	BALB/c mice	-	3 month	3 months	[29]
		Zinc Oxide NPs					[37]
Metal NPs		Albendazole-Loaded Silver NPs	Female albino mice	100 mg/kg	2 month	2 months	[38]
		Silver NPs	Female albino mice	25 mg/kg	2 month	2 months	[38]
Lipid Nanocapsules (LNCs)		Albendazole -LNCs	Female CF-1 mice	5 mg/kg	1 month	6 months	[39]
			Female CF-1 mice	5 mg/kg	1 month	8 months	[18]
		Praziquantel Loaded SLN	Female BALB/c mice	-	3 month	5 months	[40]
		Albendazole Loaded SLN	Female BALB/c mice	-	3 month	5 months	[40]
Solid lipid nanoparticles (SLNs)		Albendazole Sulfoxide Loaded SLN	Male BALB/c mice	0.5 mg/kg 2 mg/kg	15 day	8 months	[41]
		Albendazole Loaded SLN	BALB/c mice	-	-	3 months	[15]

Table 3. A list of ex vivo studies on effects of nanoparticles against hydtid cysts.

Group	Drug	Outcome		Ref
		Concentration of Drug (mL)	Best Exposure Time	
Nonmetal Nanoparticles	Albendazole Loaded NPs	0.5	-	[42]
Metal Nanoparticles	Gold NPs	0.4 0.8	- 120 min	[43]

4. Discussion

4.1. Preparation Methods of Nanoparticles

According to some factors such as condition of reaction, operation, and approved protocols, several techniques can be used for the nanoparticles synthesis. Currently, there are two main preparation methods, which include (i) bottom-up synthesis or chemo-physical methods such as lipid phase methods (precipitation, sol-gel, hydro-thermal approaches), gas phase methods (flame hydrolysis, spray hydrolysis, and aerosol methods), and biological production by plants, bacteria, fungi, etc., and (ii) top-down synthesis or mechanical-physical methods such as chemical etching, mechanical milling, sputtering, laser ablation, electro-explosion, etc. [44–46].

4.2. Solid Lipid Nanoparticles (SLNs)

SLNs have been used as a carrier system since the early 1990s. The advantages of these nanoparticles lie with their capability in drug release control, drug targeting, increasing drug chemical stability, acting as a carrier for lipophilic and hydrophilic drugs, having mass production capability, and being completely sterilized. They also increase the bioavailability of praziquantel (PZQ), enhance the pharmacological activity as well as therapeutic efficacy of PZQ and its therapeutic effect and efficacy, and reduce dose and administration frequency [15,47,48].

4.3. Albendazole (ABZ)-Loaded SLNs

In a recent study by Aminpour et al., the protoscolicidal effects of albendazole-loaded SLN (ABZ-loaded SLN) were investigated both in vitro and in vivo. In this study, during the seven-day period, the protoscoleces were exposed to the concentrations of 250 and 500 µg/mL of the drug. Then, the number of the remaining cysts was evaluated. On the fifth day of testing, all the protoscoleces in contact with ABZ-loaded SLN disappeared while protoscoleces in contact with the same concentrations of ABZ were destroyed on day 7 of the experiment. On the third day of the experiment, 5 CC of protoscoleces at the concentration of 250 µg/mL ABZ-loaded SLN was injected into the mice and, after three months, the pathogenicity of the protoscoleces in contact with the drug was investigated. It was found that in some of the mice after receiving the above compound, no cysts were formed; the remaining mice had much smaller cysts than the other groups that received ABZ only or did not receive any treatment at all. The results of this study indicated the efficient prophylactic effect of this drug on the treatment of hydatid cysts [15].

4.4. Albendazole Sulfoxide-Loaded SLNs

In a study in 2013, Ahmadnia et al. investigated the effects of albendazole sulfoxide-loaded SLN (ALBSO-loaded SLN) on hydatid cysts. The results showed this compound reduced the size of the cysts, but made no significant changes over the duration of this experiment (15 days) and still required more precise experiments, more dosing studies, and longer-term studies [41]. In another study, Soltani et al. (2015) aimed to compare hydatid cyst membrane permeability of ABZ, ABZSO, ABZ-loaded SLN, and ABZSO-loaded SLNs. Their results showed ABZ and ABZSO, due to some unique properties such as good physicochemical characterizations, controlled release, higher permeability, and efficacy by loading into SLNs, were promising for hydatid cyst treatment [17]. In a study published by Rafiei et al. (2019), ultrastructural changes of fertile and infertile cysts exposed to 2 µg/mL of ABZ-loaded SLN and ABZSO-loaded SLNs were investigated. In the histopathologic evaluation of cysts in the control group, which did not receive treatment; in this case, no structural changes were observed, while in the groups treated with the mentioned nanoparticles, the cyst structure was not integrated and only the residues and fragments of protoscoleces were present. The best performance was also observed in the ABZSO-loaded SLNs treated group [16].

4.5. Albendazole- and Praziquantile-Loaded SLNs

A 2016 study by Jelowdar et al. on PZQ- and ABZ-loaded SLNs showed that, by giving the drug to mice infected with protoscoleces, the spread of cysts in mice receiving these compounds was much lower than that in the control group receiving only SLNs without the drug. In this group of mice, there was a significant decrease in the size and dry weight of the cysts and the damaged layers of the cysts were highly observed in the mice treated with the above nanoparticles. It should be noted that in comparison to the effect of PZQ- and ABZ-loaded SLNs with free PQZ and ABZ, no significant difference was observed in the number and size of cysts; but, in the destruction rate of cyst layers in the recipient group of PZQ- and ABZ-loaded SLNs, LL loss and serious damage to GL were found. In the group receiving free ABZ and PZQ, only this layer became thin and fragile, and the number of GL cells decreased [40].

4.6. Nanolipid Carriers

This combination, created by the change in SLNs, has some advantages. These changes maintain the physical stability of the compound and facilitate the incorporation of more drug into the nanocarier. This compound has been studied in various respects and the results have shown anti-inflammatory, antimicrobial, and efficient drug delivery carriers for anti-cancer drugs [49–51].

Nanolipid Carriers-Loaded Ivermectin

In 2019, Ahmadpour et al. investigated the effect of nanolipid carriers-loaded ivermectin on the treatment of hydatid cysts. In this study, the concentrations of 200, 500, and 800 µg/mL at 150, 120, and 60 min were able to destroy hydatid cyst protoscoleces, whereas free ivermectin, at concentrations of 800 µg/mL at 150 min, was able to achieve this percentage [19].

4.7. Lipid Nanocapsules

LNCs are remarkable structures in the medical field. The benefits of this combination have led to their use not only in therapeutic applications, but also in the fields of drug delivery, cancer diagnosis, and gene and cell therapy. Studies of this compound in the field of cancer have shown promising results, indicating that this compound could reduce tumor mass and increase the cytotoxicity of glioma cells [52].

Albendazole-Lipid Nanocapsules

In 2019, Ullio Gamboa et al. investigated the protoscolicidal effects of albendazole-lipid nanocapsules (ABZ LNCs). In this study, various parameters such as LNCs drug payload and encapsulation efficiency, nanoparticle stability, stability of the nanocapsules in simulated gastrointestinal fluids, and animal studies were investigated, all of which had promising results. As seen in the animal studies, 4 out of the 10 infected mice receiving this compound showed no improvement in the cyst development and the size of the cysts decreased significantly compared to the control group. GL was also highly deformed and its cells were reduced [39]. In 2015, Pensela et al. investigated ABZ LNCs in the mice infected with hydatid cysts. In this study, we investigated the plasma and cyst drug exposure after administering ABZ as ABZ-LNCs or ABZ suspension and compared the clinical effects of these two formulations. In the studies following the use of these two formulations, ABZ levels in plasma and cysts were significantly higher when ABZ was used in combination with nanoparticles compared to ABZ suspension [18].

4.8. Metal Nanoparticles

Metallic nanoparticles are among the most efficient nanoparticles in various medical fields such as cancer therapy, respiratory disease therapy, neurodegenerative disease therapy, infectious diseases therapy, etc. [43,44]. These nanoparticles have anti-bacterial and biofilm prevention effects by producing ROS, protein adhesion, and membrane destabilization. The anti-cancer effect of these nanoparticles has also been shown to have strong effects on the cancer cells [53,54].

4.8.1. Selenium (Se) NPs

Various studies have been carried out on this nanoparticle, investigating its various aspects. In these studies, we observed a decrease in acute Se toxicity, induction of apoptosis in cancer cells, minimal side-effects on normal cells, and reduction in apoptosis in the diabetic kidney [55,56]. In evaluating the antimicrobial effects of these nanoparticles, these compounds have antimicrobial effects on methicillin-sensitive and methicillin-resistant *Staphylococcus aureus*. Antifungal and antiparasitic effects of these compounds have also been observed. These properties as well as the anti-cancer effects have made these compounds an important part of drug making [57,58].

In 2014, for the first time, the effects of biogenic selenium nanoparticles were evaluated by Mahmoudvand et al. In this study, the concentrations of 500 and 250 µg/mL of this compound for 10 and 20 min had 100% efficacy on the protoscoleces of hydatid cyst, indicating this compound had strong protoscolicidal effects [15]. In 2018, the effect of Se and Ag on the protoscoleces was evaluated by Nematollahi et al. Examining different concentrations of these compounds over 10 to 30 min showed that Se NPs were much stronger than Ag NPs and had approximately 42% yield over 60 min [20].

4.8.2. Silver (Ag) NPs

The antimicrobial and antiparasitic effects of silver nanoparticles have been studied in various studies and promising results have been obtained in cancer-related studies. The antiviral effects of silver nanoparticles have been shown to inhibit replication and binding to the host cell membrane and anti-parasitic studies have demonstrated the inhibition of proliferation and metabolic activity of promastigotes in leishmaniasis. One of the reasons that have led these nanoparticles to attract more attention is their promising effects on developing anticancer drugs [59–63].

In studies on biogenic Ag NPs by Rahimi et al. in 2015, at concentrations of 0.025, 0.05, 0.1, and 0.15 mg/mL, only the concentration of 0.15 mg/mL at 120 min was observed to have 90% protoscolicidal effects. The lowest protoscolicidal activity was also observed at 0.025 mg/mL concentration and 10 min [23]. In addition, Lashkarizadeh et al. reported this nanoparticle in the same year to have poor protoscolicidal effects on the protoscoleces of hydatid cysts, so that at concentrations of 4mg/mL for the period of 60 min, it was able to eliminate 71.6% of protoscoleces, while hypertonic salt solution at a concentration of 20% was able to eliminate 100% of protoscoleces in 10 min [22].

In a recent study by Nassef et al., the therapeutic effects of albendazole-loaded silver nanoparticles along with ABZ and Ag NPs were evaluated. These studies have shown that this compound had the highest pharmacological effect among ABZ and Ag NPs and had the least histopathological effects on the liver. In addition, in the cysts in contact with this nanoparticle, there were marked ultrastructural changes. While measuring size, granuloma size, and weight of cysts, the greatest decrease was in ABZ loaded with silver nanoparticles [38]. In a study by Norouzi et al., the protoscolicidal effects of silver, silica, copper, iron, and zinc nanoparticles were evaluated. In this in vitro work, the highest protoscolicidal effects were related to Ag-NPs at 1 mg/mL concentration after 60 min of exposure time (80% mortality rate), followed by Si-NPs at 1 mg/mL concentration (52.33%), Cu-NPs at 0.5 mg/mL concentration (41%), Fe-NPs at 1mg/mL concentration (28%), and Zn-NPs at concentration of 1mg/mL after 60 min (15.67%) [24].

4.8.3. Gold (Au) NPs

Gold nanoparticles are among the most important compounds in the medical field. There have been numerous studies on the treatment of important parasitic diseases such as leishmaniasis and malaria that have shown successful results. In addition, applying these nanoparticles for identifying different parasites has also been studied and confirmed. Gold nanoparticles have been shown to have a highly stable and adaptable structure for drug delivery, which has increased the interest in these nanoparticles [64,65].

In the recent study by Napooni on the protoscolicidal effects of this nanoparticle, we observed that the highest lethal effect was at 60-min exposure to protoscoleces with 4000 µg/mL gold nanoparticles. Furthermore, the cytotoxicity of this compound was found to be low at all concentrations. Ultrastructure changes in the tegument, shape of the sucker, size, and DNA fragmentation were also observed in protoscoleces [26]. Another study in 2016 on these nanoparticles by Barabadi et al. showed that the in vitro use of 300 µg/mL of these nanoparticles compared to other groups (groups receiving 5% normal saline and concentrations of 50, 100, and 200 µg/mL gold nanoparticles) had the highest removal rate of protoscoleces in 2 h [25]. In a recent study by Çolak et al., the protoscolicidal activity of AuNPs at concentrations of 0.4 and 0.8 mL and three laser powers including 30, 50, and 150 mW were evaluated for 30, 60, and 120 min. They found that 89.3% of the protoscoleces was killed after treatment with AuNPs under high dose (150 mW) laser power for 120 min, indicating that increasing the dose of AuNPs or laser power or used time increased the mortality rate of protoscoleces [43].

Malekifard et al. (2017) also investigated the protoscolicidal effects of these nanoparticles. Protoscolicidal effects of gold nanoparticles were studied in vitro at concentrations of 250, 500, and 1000 µg/mL for 5 to 60 min in contact with hydatid cyst fluid. Gold nanoparticles at all concentrations used had significant protoscolicidal effects compared to the control group, so that all the protoscoleces in contact with the concentration of 1000 µg/mL were eliminated within 1 h [27].

4.9. Non-Metal NPs

ABZ-Loaded Nanoparticles

In a study in 2008, Truong Cong et al. evaluated the diffusion ability of ABZ nanoparticles and increased drug concentration in hydatid cysts. A good correlation was observed between the permeation coefficient and partition coefficient. The drug release from the nanoparticles through the hydatid membrane was improved compared to the soluble ABZ and showed sufficient entrapment efficiency to increase the apparent solubility of ABZ [42].

4.10. Metal Oxide NPs

4.10.1. Zinc Oxide Nanoparticles

ZnO nanoparticles are non-toxic and compatible with body skin. Properties such as skin adaptation, non-toxicity, antimicrobial, antiparasitic, and antifungal activity have made these nanoparticles a widely-used and important compound in manufacturing medicine. These nanoparticles, without toxic effects on healthy cells, induce death in cancer cells; studies have shown that these nanoparticles can be used for gene delivery [66,67].

Norouzi et al. recently investigated the protoscolicidal effects of zinc oxide nanoparticles for the first time. At 50 and 100 mg/mL concentrations, the highest protoscolicidal effects of this compound were observed in 10 min of zinc oxide and protoscolece nanoparticles exposure, which was 19.6% (very weak) and with no increase in performance over time; it was a low percentage, indicating this compound was not suitable for use in hydatid cyst surgery [28]. In another study on this nanoparticle in 2015 by Razi Jalali et al., the protoscolicidal effects of zinc oxide and ABZ, *Echinacea purpurea*, and *Sambucus ebulus* nanoparticles were investigated, which revealed a decrease in size, volume, and number of cysts in all the compounds [37].

4.10.2. Titanium Dioxide (TiO2) Nanoparticles

TiO2 nanoparticles are considered as one of the most widely used nanoparticles in various industries such as cosmetics, food, and pharmaceuticals, since they have some physicochemical properties such as non-toxicity, cost-effectiveness, anticorrosive, high stability, photocatalytic properties, etc. These compounds kill cells by inactivating germ cell and DNA enzymes as well as by removing fluids from bacterial cells. Other uses of these compounds include treating and diagnosing cancer [68–70]. Navvabi et al. (2019) recently investigated the in vitro and in viovo protoscolicidal effects of *Echinometra mathaei* (sea urchin gonad) extract alone or combined with TiO2 NPs. Their results showed that sea urchin gonad extract at the concentration 15 μg/mL, especially in combination with TiO2, killed 84% of the protoscoleces after 60 min exposure in vitro. On the other hand, oral administration of infected mice with the combination of the gonad extract + TiO2 for three months demonstrated higher efficacy by reduction in number, size and volume of the hydatid cysts in comparison to the control group [29].

4.10.3. Cerium Dioxide Nanoparticles

Cerium (Ce) is one of the rare-earth elements that, because of its special structure, has expended its use. Other features include its cost-effectiveness. Many studies have investigated the benefits of this nanoparticle, such as antimicrobial, anti-cancer, treatment, and antioxidant activities [71,72]. In a study by Aryamand et al. (2019), the in vitro and in vivo protoscolicidal effects of *Holothuria leucospilota* extract alone, CeO2 nanoparticles alone, and extract combined with CeO2 NPs were investigated for 10 to 60 min. In vitro results showed that the most protoscolicidal effects were reported for extract (70% at 20 mg/mL for 60 min), followed by the combination of this extract and Ce nanoparticles (63% in 15 mg/mL concentration for 1 h). Furthermore, in vivo assay demonstrated that all three compounds significantly reduced the number and size of the hydatid cysts compared to the control group that received no treatment [30].

4.10.4. Zirconium Dioxide Nanoparticles

Zirconium (Zr) is a chemical element which has some applications, especially in medicine and dentistry [73]. Zirconium dioxide (ZrO2), also called zirconia, has some unique properties such as high compatibility, low toxicity, low cost, and high strength and is broadly used in various biomedical fields including antimicrobial ones [74–77]. In a study conducted by Ibrahim (2020), ZrO2 at concentrations of 1000, 2000, and 4000 μg/mL significantly killed 49.6, 52.7, and 53.1% of the hydatid protoscoleces after 60 min [31].

4.11. Nanopolymeric Particles

Various properties of chitosan nanoparticles (Ch NPs) including non-toxicity, water solubility, stability, simple preparation, environmental compliance, and antimicrobial activity have made them remarkable and effective compounds in the field of medicine. In the field of vaccine development, several studies have been performed to evaluate the usefulness of these nanoparticles, showing their beneficial effects [78–80].

4.11.1. Chitosan-Curcumin Nanoparticles

In another study by Napooni et al. (2019), the in vitro protoscolicidal effects of chitosan–curcumin nanoparticle (Ch-Cu NPs) at different concentrations of 0.25, 0.05, 1, 2, and 4 mg/mL were evaluated for 5, 10, 20, 30, and 60 min. The results showed that the highest mortality rate (68%) of protoscoleces was observed after exposure to Ch-Cu-NPs at a concentration of 4000 μg/mL for 60 min, whereas by scanning electron microscopy, the length and width of protoscoleces were significantly reduced compared to the control group [32].

4.11.2. Chitosan-Praziquantel and -Albendazole Nanoparticles

Torabi et al. (2018) examined the protoscolicidal, prophylactic, and therapeutic effects of ChPZQ and ChABZ. In evaluating the in vitro protoscolicidal effects of these compounds, microcysts were exposed (for 16 days) at concentrations of 1, 5, and 10 µg/mL of chitosan-praziquantel (ChPZQ) and -albendazole (ChABZ); then, it was observed that the best effect during this time was related to using these two compounds together (at concentrations 5 and 10) when no microcysts were observed for 10 days post-incubation. Compared to ChPZQ and ChABZ, ChPZQ performed better at all the three concentrations than ChABZ (no significant difference). In order to evaluate the therapeutic and prophylactic effects of these compounds, the number and weight of cysts in contact with the above compounds were evaluated. For evaluating the prophylactic effect of these compounds, a significant decrease in the number and weight of cysts in the group receiving the two compounds was observed compared to the control group receiving no medication. However, in the evaluation of therapeutic effect, there was a significant difference in the number of cysts in the group receiving ChABZ and ChPZQ nanoparticles together compared to the control group; but no significant decrease was observed in the weight of the cysts compared to the control group. In the mice receiving both combinations, GL and LL were separated [81]. Furthermore, in another study by Torabi et al., ChPZQ showed more stability than ChABZ, which could be due to its better performance [66].

In a recent study conducted by Darvishi et al. (2020), the effects of ABZ-sulfoxide (SO)-loaded chitosan (CS)-PGLA NPs synthesized by nanoprecipitation orally administered at a dose of 10 mg/kg/day for 45 days showed significant therapeutic effect in the weight and volume of cysts in comparison to that in the control group, indicating that ABZ-SO-loaded CS-PGLA NPs could improve the therapeutic effects of ABZ-SO in the CE treatment in mice [36].

4.11.3. Albendazole Sulfoxide-Loaded PLGA-PEG NPs

In 2016, Naseri et al. investigated the protoscolicidal effects and apoptotic activity of albendazole sulfoxide-loaded PLGA-PEG (ABZs-loaded PLGA-PEG). In this study, concentrations of 50, 100, 150, and 200 µg/mL of these compounds were exposed to a specific concentration of hydatid cyst fluid for 5 to 60 min. To evaluate the protoscolicidal effects, it was observed that at concentrations of 150 and 200 µg/mL, the nanodrug (at all times of the experiment) had 100% protoscolicidal effects, while at a concentration of 200 µg/mL, albendazole at 30 min had a 100% effect. Protoscoleces treated with ABZs-loaded PLGA-PEG showed surface shrinkage, disoriented appearance, and a disrupted characteristic due to programmed cell death. Both compounds had apoptotic intensity, but no significant difference was observed in the activity of both compounds [34].

4.11.4. Flubendazole-Loaded mPEG-PCL NPs

In 2018, studies on the protoscolicidal effects of flubendazole-loaded mPEG-PCL NPs were conducted by Farhadi et al. The in vitro study showed that, at exposure time of 27 days, 10 µg/mL of these nanoparticles was able to kill all the protoscoleces on the 15th day. In vivo studies also showed that the number of cysts was significantly lower than the control group, but the difference in the number of cysts in the free flobendazole recipient group and the group that received nanoparticle was not significant. The weight of the cysts in the nanoparticle receiving group was much lower than the other groups; the cysts underwent many changes and there were marked ultrastructural changes in the germinal layer [35].

5. Conclusions

The results of this review study show the high efficacy of a wide range of organic and inorganic NPs against CE, indicating that nanoparticles could be considered as an alternative and complementary resource for CE treatment. The results demonstrated that the most widely used nanoparticles for hydatid cyst treatment are metal nanoparticles, metal oxide nanoparticles, followed by polymeric nanoparticles. We found that the most compatible drugs with nanoparticles were albendazole, followed by praziquantel and flubendazole, indicating a deeper understanding about the synergistic effects of nanoparticles and the present anti-parasitic drugs to treat hydatid cysts. The important point about using these nanoparticles is their toxicity; therefore, cytotoxicity as well as acute and chronic toxicities of these nanoparticles should be considered in particular. As a limitation, in the present study, although most studies have been performed in vitro, more studies are needed to confirm the effect of these nanoparticles as well as their exact mechanisms in hydatid cyst treatment, especially in animal models and clinical settings.

Author Contributions: A.E.A. and H.M. conceived and designed the study; M.S. and A.D.A. collected data and critical review; P.B. analyzed the data; H.M. and A.E.A. wrote the paper. All authors have read and agreed to the published version of the manuscript.

Funding: This research received no external funding.

Conflicts of Interest: The authors declare that they have no competing interests.

Availability of Data and Materials: All data generated or analyzed during this study are included in this published article.

References

1. Mcmanus, D.P.; Zhang, W.; Li, J.; Bartley, P.B. Echinococcosis. *Lancet* **2003**, *362*, 1295–1304. [CrossRef]
2. Eckert, J.; Deplazes, P. Biological, Epidemiological, and Clinical Aspects of Echinococcosis, a Zoonosis of Increasing Concern. *Clin. Microbiol. Rev.* **2004**, *17*, 107–135. [CrossRef] [PubMed]
3. Brunetti, E.; Kern, P.; Vuitton, D.A. Expert consensus for the diagnosis and treatment of cystic and alveolar echinococcosis in humans. *Acta Trop.* **2010**, *114*, 1–16. [CrossRef] [PubMed]
4. Junghanss, T.; Da Silva, A.M.; Horton, J.; Chiodini, P.L.; Brunetti, E. Clinical management of cystic echinococcosis: State of the art, problems, and perspectives. *Am. J. Trop. Med. Hyg.* **2008**, *79*, 301–311. [CrossRef]
5. Eckert, J. Guidelines for treatment of cystic and alveolar echinococcosis in humans. *Bull. World Health Organ.* **1996**, *74*, 231–242.
6. Dehkordi, A.B.; Sanei, B.; Yousefi, M.; Sharafi, S.M.; Safarnezhad, F.; Jafari, R.; Darani, H.Y. Albendazole and treatment of hydatid cyst, review of literature. *Infect. Disord. Drug Targets* **2018**, *18*, 1. [CrossRef]
7. Sahin, M.; Eryilmaz, R.; Bulbuloglu, E. The Effect of Scolicidal Agents on Liver and Biliary Tree (Experimental Study). *J. Investig. Surg.* **2004**, *17*, 323–326. [CrossRef]
8. Mishra, S. Nanotechnology in medicine. *Indian Heart J.* **2016**, *68*, 437–439. [CrossRef]
9. Zhu, X.; Radovic-Moreno, A.F.; Wu, J.; Langer, R.; Shi, J. Nanomedicine in the management of microbial infection—Overview and perspectives. *Nano Today* **2014**, *9*, 478–498. [CrossRef]
10. Sengul, A.B.; Asmatulu, E. Toxicity of metal and metal oxide nanoparticles: A review. *Environ. Chem. Lett.* **2020**, *18*, 1659–1683. [CrossRef]
11. Salata, O.V. Applications of nanoparticles in biology and medicine. *J. Nanobiotechnol.* **2004**, *2*, 3. [CrossRef]
12. Rajput, N. Methods of preparation of nanoparticles—A review. *Int. J. Adv. Eng. Technol.* **2015**, *7*, 1806.
13. Shnawa, B.H. Advances in the Use of Nanoparticles as Anti-Cystic Echinococcosis Agents: A Review Article. *J. Pharm. Res. Int.* **2018**, *24*, 1–14. [CrossRef]
14. Moher, D.; Liberati, A.; Tetzlaff, J.; Altman, D.G.; Prisma Group. Preferred reporting items for systematic reviews and meta-analyses: The PRISMA statement. *PLoS Med.* **2009**, *6*, e1000097. [CrossRef]
15. Aminpour, S.; Rafiei, A.; Jelowdar, A.; Kouchak, M. Evaluation of the Protoscolicidal Effects of Albendazole and Albendazole Loaded Solid Lipid Nanoparticles. *Iran. J. Parasitol.* **2019**, *14*, 127–135. [CrossRef]
16. Rafiei, A.; Soltani, S.; Ramezani, Z.; Abbaspour, M.R.; Jelowdar, A.; Kahvaz, M.S. Ultrastructural changes on fertile and infertile hydatid cysts induced by conventional and solid lipid nanoparticles of albendazole and albendazole sulfoxide. *Comp. Clin Path.* **2019**, *28*, 1045–1053. [CrossRef]
17. Soltani, S.; Rafiei, A.; Ramezani, Z.; Abbaspour, M.R.; Jelowdar, A.; Kahvaz, M.S. Evaluation of the hydatid cyst membrane permeability of albendazole and albendazole sulfoxide-loaded solid lipid nanoparticles. *Jundishapur J. Nat. Pharm. Prod.* **2017**, *12*, e34723.

18. Pensel, P.E.; Gamboa, G.V.U.; Fabbri, J.; Ceballos, L.; Bruni, S.S.; Alvarez, L.I.; A Allemandi, D.; Benoît, J.; Palma, S.D.; Elissondo, M.C. Cystic echinococcosis therapy: Albendazole-loaded lipid nanocapsules enhance the oral bioavailability and efficacy in experimentally infected mice. *Acta Trop.* **2015**, *152*, 185–194. [CrossRef]
19. Ahmadpour, E.; Godrati-Azar, Z.; Spotin, A.; Norouzi, R.; Hamishehkar, H.; Nami, S.; Heydarian, P.; Rajabi, S.; Mohammadi, M.; Perez-Cordon, G. Nanostructured lipid carriers of ivermectin as a novel drug delivery system in hydatidosis. *Parasites Vectors* **2019**, *12*, 1–9. [CrossRef]
20. Mahmoudvand, H.; Harandi, M.F.; Shakibaie, M.; Aflatoonian, M.R.; Zia Ali, N.; Makki, M.S.; Jahanbakhsh, S. Scolicidal effects of biogenic selenium nanoparticles against protoscoleces of hydatid cysts. *Int. J. Surg.* **2014**, *12*, 399–403. [CrossRef]
21. Nematollahi, A.; Shahbazi, P.; Rafat, A.; Ghanbarlu, M. Comparative survey on scolicidal effects of selenium and silver nanoparticles on protoscoleces of hydatid cyst. *Open Vet. J.* **2018**, *8*, 374. [CrossRef] [PubMed]
22. Lashkarizadeh, M.R.; Asgaripour, K.; Dezaki, E.S.; Harandi, M.F. Comparison of Scolicidal Effects of Amphotricin B, Silver Nanoparticles, and Foeniculum vulgare Mill on Hydatid Cysts Protoscoleces. *Iran. J. Parasitol.* **2015**, *10*, 206–212.
23. Rahimi, M.T.; Ahmadpour, E.; Esboei, B.R.; Spotin, A.; Koshki, M.H.K.; Alizadeh, A.; Honary, S.; Barabadi, H.; Mohammadi, M.A. Scolicidal activity of biosynthesized silver nanoparticles against Echinococcus granulosus protoscoleces. *Int. J. Surg.* **2015**, *19*, 128–133. [CrossRef]
24. Norouzi, R.; Ataei, A.; Hejazy, M.; Noreddin, A.; Ezzat, M.; Zowalaty, E. Scolicidal Effects of Nanoparticles Against Hydatid Cyst Protoscoleces in vitro. *Int. J. Nanomed.* **2020**, *15*, 1095. [CrossRef] [PubMed]
25. Barabadi, H.; Honary, S.; Ali Mohammadi, M.; Ahmadpour, E.; Rahimi, M.T.; Alizadeh, A.; Naghibi, F.; Saravanan, M. Green chemical synthesis of gold nanoparticles by using Penicillium aculeatum and their scolicidal activity against hydatid cyst protoscoleces of Echinococcus granulosus. *Environ. Sci. Pollut. Res.* **2017**, *24*, 5800–5810. [CrossRef] [PubMed]
26. Napooni, S.; Arbabi, M.; Delavari, M.; Hooshyar, H.; Rasti, S. Lethal effects of gold nanoparticles on protoscoleces of hydatid cyst: In vitro study. *Comp. Clin. Path.* **2019**, *28*, 143–150. [CrossRef]
27. Malekifard, F. Solicidal effect of the gold nanoparticle on protoscoleces of hydratid cyst in vitro. *J. URMIA Univ. Med. Sci.* **2017**, *28*, 137.
28. Norouzi, R.; Hejazy, M.; Ataei, A. Scolicidal effect of zinc oxide nanoparticles against hydatid cyst protoscoleces in vitro. *Int. J. Nanomed.* **2019**, *4*, 23–28.
29. Navvabi, A.; Homaei, A.; Khademvatan, S.; Ansari, M.H.K.; Keshavarz, M. Combination of TiO_2 nanoparticles and Echinometra mathaeis gonad extracts: In vitro and in vivo scolicidal activity against hydatid cysts. *Biocatal. Agric. Biotechnol.* **2019**, *22*, 101432. [CrossRef]
30. Aryamand, S.; Khademvatan, S.; Tappeh, K.H.; Heshmatian, B.; Jelodar, A. In Vitro and in Vivo Scolicidal Activities of Holothuria leucospilota Extract and CeO_2 Nanoparticles against Hydatid Cyst. *Iran. J. Parasitol.* **2019**, *14*, 269–279. [CrossRef]
31. Ibrahim, A.A.J. Scolicidal Activity of Zirconium Oxide (ZrO_2) nanoparticles Against Protoscolices of Hydatid Cysts. *Indian J. Forensic Med. Toxicol.* **2020**, *14*, 409.
32. Napooni, S.; Delavari, M.; Arbabi, M.; Barkheh, H.; Rasti, S.; Hooshyar, H.; Mashkani, S.M.H. Scolicidal Effects of Chitosan–Curcumin Nanoparticles on the Hydatid Cyst Protoscoleces. *Acta Parasitol.* **2019**, *64*, 367–375. [CrossRef] [PubMed]
33. Torabi, N.; Dobakhti, F.; Faghihzadeh, S.; Haniloo, A. In vitro and in vivo effects of chitosan-praziquantel and chitosan-albendazole nanoparticles on Echinococcus granulosus Metacestodes. *Parasitol. Res.* **2018**, *117*, 2015–2023. [CrossRef]
34. Naseri, M.; Akbarzadeh, A.; Spotin, A.; Akbari, N.A.R.; Mahami-Oskouei, M.; Ahmadpour, E. Scolicidal and apoptotic activities of albendazole sulfoxide and albendazole sulfoxide-loaded PLGA-PEG as a novel nanopolymeric particle against Echinococcus granulosus protoscoleces. *Parasitol. Res.* **2016**, *115*, 4595–4603. [CrossRef] [PubMed]
35. Farhadi, M.; Haniloo, A.; Rostamizadeh, K.; Faghihzadeh, S. Efficiency of flubendazole-loaded mPEG-PCL nanoparticles: A promising formulation against the protoscoleces and cysts of Echinococcus granulosus. *Acta Trop.* **2018**, *187*, 190–200. [CrossRef] [PubMed]
36. Darvishi, M.M.; Moazeni, M.; Alizadeh, M.; Abedi, M.; Tamaddon, A.-M. Evaluation of the efficacy of albendazole sulfoxide (ABZ-SO)–loaded chitosan-PLGA nanoparticles in the treatment of cystic echinococcosis in laboratory mice. *Parasitol. Res.* **2020**, *119*, 4233–4241. [CrossRef] [PubMed]

37. Razi, J.M.; Alborzi, A.; Najafzade Varzi, H.; Ghorbanpour, M.; Derakhshan, L. Survey on effects of albendazole, echinacea purpurea, sambucus ebulus and zinc oxide nanoparticles on unilocular hydatid cyst in mice. *Sci. Iran. Vet. J.* **2015**, *11*, 68–125.
38. Nassef, N.E.; Saad, A.-G.E.; Harba, N.M.; Beshay, E.V.N.; Gouda, M.A.; Shendi, S.S.; Mohamed, A.S.E.-D. Evaluation of the therapeutic efficacy of albendazole-loaded silver nanoparticles against Echinococcus granulosus infection in experimental mice. *J. Parasit. Dis.* **2019**, *43*, 658–671. [CrossRef]
39. Gamboa, G.V.U.; Pensel, P.E.; Elissondo, M.C.; Bruni, S.F.S.; Benoît, J.; Palma, S.D.; Allemandi, A. Albendazole-lipid nanocapsules: Optimization, characterization and chemoprophylactic efficacy in mice infected with Echinococcus granulosus. *Exp. Parasitol.* **2019**, *198*, 79–86. [CrossRef]
40. Jelowdar, A.; Rafiei, A.; Abbaspour, M.; Rashidi, I.; Rahdar, M. Efficacy of combined albendazol and praziquntel and their loaded solid lipid nanoparticles components in chemoprophylaxis of experimental hydatidosis. *Asian Pac. J. Trop. Biomed.* **2017**, *7*, 549–554. [CrossRef]
41. Ahmadnia, S.; Moazeni, M.; Mohammadi-Samani, S.; Oryan, A. In vivo evaluation of the efficacy of albendazole sulfoxide and albendazole sulfoxide loaded solid lipid nanoparticles against hydatid cyst. *Exp. Parasitol.* **2013**, *135*, 314–319. [CrossRef] [PubMed]
42. Cong, T.T.; Faivre, V.; Nguyen, T.T.; Heras, H.; Pirot, F.; Walchshofer, N.; Sarciron, M.-E.; Falson, F. Study on the hydatid cyst membrane: Permeation of model molecules and interactions with drug-loaded nanoparticles. *Int. J. Pharm.* **2008**, *353*, 223–232. [CrossRef]
43. Çolak, B.; Aksoy, F.; Yavuz, S.; Demircili, M.E. Investigating the effect of gold nanoparticles on hydatid cyst protoscoleces under low-power green laser irradiation. *Turk. J. Surg.* **2019**, *35*, 314–320. [CrossRef] [PubMed]
44. Okuyama, K.; Lenggoro, I.W. Preparation of nanoparticles via spray route. *Chem. Eng. Sci.* **2003**, *58*, 537–547. [CrossRef]
45. Jahn, A.; Reiner, J.E.; Vreeland, W.N.; DeVoe, D.L.; Locascio, L.E.; Gaitan, M. Preparation of nanoparticles by continuous-flow microfluidics. *J. Nanoparticle. Res.* **2008**, *10*, 925–934. [CrossRef]
46. Khan, I.; Saeed, K.; Khan, I. Nanoparticles: Properties, applications and toxicities. *Arab. J. Chem.* **2019**, *12*, 908–931. [CrossRef]
47. Li, Y.; Yehui, G.; Hao, L.; Yu, Z.; Jinsong, Y.; Yanyan, C. Enhancement the oral bioavailability of praziquantel by incorporation into solid lipid nanoparticles. *Pharmazie* **2009**, *64*, 86–89.
48. Xie, S.; Pan, B.; Shi, B.; Zhang, Z.; Zhang, X.; Wang, M.; Zhou, W. Solid lipid nanoparticle suspension enhanced the therapeutic efficacy of praziquantel against tapeworm. *Int. J. Nanomed.* **2011**, *6*, 2367–2374. [CrossRef]
49. Purohit, D.K.; Nandgude, T.D.; Poddar, S.S. Nano-lipid carriers for topical application: Current scenario. *Asian J. Pharm.* **2016**, *10*, S1–S9.
50. Beloqui, A.; Solinís, M.Á.; Rodríguez-Gascón, A.; Almeida, A.J.; Préat, V. Nanostructured lipid carriers: Promising drug delivery systems for future clinics. *Nanomed. Nanotechnol. Biol. Med.* **2016**, *12*, 143–161. [CrossRef]
51. Cortesi, R.; Valacchi, G.; Muresan, X.M.; Drechsler, M.; Contado, C.; Esposito, E.; Grandini, A.; Guerrini, A.; Forlani, G.; Sacchetti, G. Nanostructured lipid carriers (NLC) for the delivery of natural molecules with antimicrobial activity: Production, characterisation and in vitro studies. *J. Microencapsul.* **2017**, *34*, 63–72. [CrossRef] [PubMed]
52. Huynh, N.; Passirani, C.; Saulnier, P.; Benoit, J.P. Lipid nanocapsules: A new platform for nanomedicine. *Int. J. Pharm.* **2009**, *379*, 201–209. [CrossRef] [PubMed]
53. Conde, J.; Doria, G.; Baptista, P. Noble Metal Nanoparticles Applications in Cancer. *J. Drug Deliv.* **2012**, *2012*, 1–12. [CrossRef] [PubMed]
54. Gold, K.; Slay, B.; Knackstedt, M.; Gaharwar, A.K. Antimicrobial Activity of Metal and Metal-Oxide Based Nanoparticles. *Adv. Ther.* **2018**, *1*. [CrossRef]
55. Kumar, G.S.; Kulkarni, A.; Khurana, A.; Kaur, J.; Tikoo, K. Selenium nanoparticles involve HSP-70 and SIRT1 in preventing the progression of type 1 diabetic nephropathy. *Chem. Biol. Interact.* **2014**, *223*, 125–133. [CrossRef]
56. Khurana, A.; Tekula, S.; Saifi, M.A.; Venkatesh, P.; Godugu, C. Therapeutic applications of selenium nanoparticles. *Biomed. Pharmacother.* **2019**, *111*, 802–812. [CrossRef]

57. Wadhwani, S.A.; Shedbalkar, U.U.; Singh, R.; Chopade, B.A. Biogenic selenium nanoparticles: Current status and future prospects. *Appl. Microbiol. Biotechnol.* **2016**, *100*, 2555–2566. [CrossRef]
58. Huang, T.; Holden, J.A.; Heath, D.E.; O'Brien-Simpson, N.M.; O'Connor, A.J. Engineering highly effective antimicrobial selenium nanoparticles through control of particle size. *Nanoscale* **2019**, *11*, 14937–14951. [CrossRef]
59. Wei, L.; Lu, J.; Xu, H.; Patel, A.; Chen, Z.-S.; Chen, G. Silver nanoparticles: Synthesis, properties, and therapeutic applications. *Drug Discov. Today* **2015**, *20*, 595–601. [CrossRef]
60. Gaafar, M.R.; Mady, R.; Diab, R.; Shalaby, T. Chitosan and silver nanoparticles: Promising anti-toxoplasma agents. *Exp. Parasitol.* **2014**, *143*, 30–38. [CrossRef]
61. Allahverdiyev, A.; Abamor, E.Ş.; Bagirova, M.; Ustundag, C.B.; Kaya, C.; Rafailovich, M. Antileishmanial effect of silver nanoparticles and their enhanced antiparasitic activity under ultraviolet light. *Int. J. Nanomed.* **2011**, *6*, 2705–2714. [CrossRef] [PubMed]
62. Galdiero, S.; Falanga, A.; Vitiello, M.; Cantisani, M.; Marra, V.; Galdiero, M. Silver Nanoparticles as Potential Antiviral Agents. *Molecules* **2011**, *16*, 8894–8918. [CrossRef] [PubMed]
63. Dos Santos, C.A.; Rai, M.; Ingle, A.P.; Gupta, I.; Galdiero, S.; Galdiero, M.; Gade, A.; Rai, M. Silver Nanoparticles: Therapeutical Uses, Toxicity, and Safety Issues. *J. Pharm. Sci.* **2014**, *103*, 1931–1944. [CrossRef] [PubMed]
64. Thambiraj, S.; Hema, S.; Shankaran, D.R. Functionalized gold nanoparticles for drug delivery applications. *Mater. Today Proc.* **2018**, *5*, 16763–16773. [CrossRef]
65. Benelli, G. Gold nanoparticles—Against parasites and insect vectors. *Acta Trop.* **2018**, *178*, 73–80. [CrossRef]
66. Webster, T.J.T.; Taylor, E. Reducing infections through nanotechnology and nanoparticles. *Int. J. Nanomed.* **2011**, *6*, 1463–1473. [CrossRef]
67. Mirzaei, H.; Darroudi, M. Zinc oxide nanoparticles: Biological synthesis and biomedical applications. *Ceram. Int.* **2017**, *43*, 907–914. [CrossRef]
68. Çeşmeli, S.; Avci, C.B. Application of titanium dioxide (TiO$_2$) nanoparticles in cancer therapies. *J. Drug Target.* **2019**, *27*, 762–766. [CrossRef]
69. Alhadrami, H.A.; Baqasi, A.; Iqbal, J.; Shoudri, R.A.; Ashshi, A.M.; Azhar, E.I.; Al-Hazmi, F.; Al-Ghamdi, A.; Wageh, S. Antibacterial Applications of Anatase TiO$_2$ Nanoparticle. *Am. J. Nanomater.* **2017**, *5*, 31–42. [CrossRef]
70. Peiris, M.M.K.; Guansekera, T.D.C.P.; Jayaweera, P.M.; Fernando, S.S.N. TiO$_2$ nanoparticles from baker's yeast: A potent antimicrobial. *J. Microbiol. Biotechnol.* **2018**, *28*, 1664–1670. [CrossRef]
71. Dhall, A.; Self, W.T. Cerium Oxide Nanoparticles: A Brief Review of Their Synthesis Methods and Biomedical Applications. *Antioxidants* **2018**, *7*, 97. [CrossRef] [PubMed]
72. Nithya, P.; Sundrarajan, M. Ionic liquid functionalized biogenic synthesis of Ag[sbnd]Au bimetal doped CeO$_2$ nanoparticles from Justicia adhatoda for pharmaceutical applications: Antibacterial and anti-cancer activities. *J. Photochem. Photobiol. B Biol.* **2020**, *202*, 111706. [CrossRef] [PubMed]
73. Chen, Y.-W.; Moussi, J.; Drury, J.L.; Wataha, J.C. Zirconia in biomedical applications. *Expert Rev. Med. Devices* **2016**, *13*, 945–963. [CrossRef] [PubMed]
74. Larsson, C. Zirconium dioxide based dental restorations. Studies on clinical performance and fracture behaviour. *Swed. Dent. J. Suppl.* **2011**, *213*, 9.
75. Patil, N.A.; Kandasubramanian, B. Biological and mechanical enhancement of zirconium dioxide for medical applications. *Ceram. Int.* **2020**, *46*, 4041–4057. [CrossRef]
76. Fathima, J.B.; Pugazhendhi, A.; Venis, R. Synthesis and characterization of ZrO$_2$ nanoparticles-antimicrobial activity and their prospective role in dental care. *Microb. Pathog.* **2017**, *110*, 245–251. [CrossRef] [PubMed]
77. Gowri, S.; Gandhi, R.R.; Sundrarajan, M. Structural, Optical, Antibacterial and Antifungal Properties of Zirconia Nanoparticles by Biobased Protocol. *J. Mater. Sci. Technol.* **2014**, *30*, 782–790. [CrossRef]
78. Tiyabooncjai, W.; Tiyaboonchai, W. Chitosan nanoparticles: A promising system for drug delivery. *Naresuan Univ. J.* **2003**, *3*, 51–66.
79. Illum, L.; Jabbal-Gill, I.; Hinchcliffe, M.; Fisher, A.; Davis, S. Chitosan as a novel nasal delivery system for vaccines. *Adv. Drug Deliv. Rev.* **2001**, *51*, 81–96. [CrossRef]

80. Divya, K.; Jisha, M. Chitosan nanoparticles preparation and applications. *Environ. Chem. Lett.* **2018**, *16*, 101–112. [CrossRef]
81. Torabi, N.; Dobakhti, F.; Haniloo, A. Albendazole and Praziquantel Chitosan Nanoparticles: Preparation, Characterization, and In Vitro Release Study. *Iran. J. Sci. Technol. Trans. A Sci.* **2018**, *42*, 1269–1275. [CrossRef]

Publisher's Note: MDPI stays neutral with regard to jurisdictional claims in published maps and institutional affiliations.

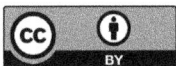

© 2020 by the authors. Licensee MDPI, Basel, Switzerland. This article is an open access article distributed under the terms and conditions of the Creative Commons Attribution (CC BY) license (http://creativecommons.org/licenses/by/4.0/).

MDPI
St. Alban-Anlage 66
4052 Basel
Switzerland
Tel. +41 61 683 77 34
Fax +41 61 302 89 18
www.mdpi.com

Nanomaterials Editorial Office
E-mail: nanomaterials@mdpi.com
www.mdpi.com/journal/nanomaterials

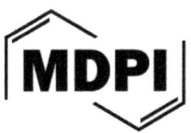